MW01247800

Raising NATHAN
AGAINST ALL ODDS

DISCOVERING THE BLESSINGS, JOY, AND
PURPOSE IN RAISING A CHILD
WITH DISABILITIES

CHRISTINE E. STAPLE EBANKS
FOREWORD BY SENTA GREENE

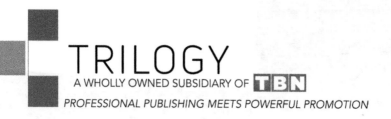

Trilogy Christian Publishers

A Wholly Owned Subsidary of Trinity Broadcasting Network

2442 Michelle Drive

Tustin, CA 92780

Copyright © 2024 by Christine E. Staple Ebanks

Scripture quotations marked NIV are taken from the Holy Bible, New International Version®, NIV®. Copyright © 1973, 1978, 1984, 2011 by Biblica, Inc.TM Used by permission of Zondervan. All rights reserved worldwide. www.zondervan.com. The "NIV" and "New International Version" are trademarks registered in the United States Patent and Trademark Office by Biblica, Inc.TM. Scripture quotations marked NKJV are taken from the New King James Version®. Copyright © 1982 by Thomas Nelson. Used by permission. All rights reserved.

All rights reserved, including the right to reproduce this book or portions thereof in any form whatsoever.

For information, address Trilogy Christian Publishing

Rights Department, 2442 Michelle Drive, Tustin, Ca 92780.

Trilogy Christian Publishing/ TBN and colophon are trademarks of Trinity Broadcasting Network.

For information about special discounts for bulk purchases, please contact Trilogy Christian Publishing.

Trilogy Disclaimer: The views and content expressed in this book are those of the author and may not necessarily reflect the views and doctrine of Trilogy Christian Publishing or the Trinity Broadcasting Network.

10 9 8 7 6 5 4 3 2 1

Library of Congress Cataloging-in-Publication Data is available.

ISBN 979-8-89041-792-3

ISBN 979-8-89041-793-0 (ebook)

"The stone the builders rejected has become the cornerstone."

Psalm 118:22 (NIV)

DEDICATION

In loving memory of Ryman and Ivy Ebanks,
and Dawn Coombs

Our children with disabilities are not defined by their limitations; they are defined by the boundless love and purpose they bring into our lives.

—Unknown

ACKNOWLEDGMENTS

When a child has a disability, its impact extends far beyond the individual's special needs; it ripples through the lives of everyone who loves, cares for, and supports them. This journey leaves an indelible mark on the entire family, from parents and siblings to grandparents, aunts, uncles, and cousins. It extends into the broader community, encompassing friends, educators, therapists, doctors, and countless others who become integral threads in this intricate tapestry woven with faith, compassion, love, patience, and unwavering perseverance. Much like the journey of raising Nathan, writing *Raising Nathan Against All Odds: Discovering the Blessings, Joy, and Purpose in Raising a Child with Disabilities* has been a labor of love—a testament to this faithful and supportive community.

First and foremost, my deepest gratitude goes to God, the author and finisher of my faith, for the countless blessings He bestowed upon our lives through the gift of Nathan. It is through the transformative experience of raising him that I gained a true understanding of this road less traveled of raising a child with disabilities. It is the very experience that ignited my compassion and determination to make a meaningful difference for other families facing similar journeys.

I want to express my deepest appreciation to my beloved family. To my husband and best friend, Robert, your commitment to our family, steadfast encouragement, and belief in this project have been my rock. To my children, Adrianne, Ryan, Jordanne, and Nathan, your unique perspectives and constant love have enriched this story beyond measure. Thank you for being an integral part of this narrative and for helping me see the world through your eyes. Your support during this writing process, taking over aspects of our daily lives at times, and the laughter and hugs that kept me going mean more to me than words can express.

To Ryman and Ivy Ebanks' blessed memory. You taught me the power of love and the blessings of grandparents. Your support of Nathan and our family knows no measure. Thank you for your prayers. To my dear mother, Aleith, your constant encouragement and prayers have guided us throughout this journey. To my sisters, Jennifer and Phyllis, and other siblings who have contributed to our lives at one point or another, your support and sisterly love have meant the world to me.

I am profoundly grateful to the incredible contributors who have played vital roles in the creation of this book. Erin Mercer, your friendship, exceptional developmental editing, and empathetic support were indispensable while revisiting and confronting some of the more painful aspects of my experience. Senta Greene, thank you for crafting a moving foreword that sets the tone for this book and captures its essence with such grace and eloquence. For more than a decade, your steadfast partnership in nurturing hope has firmly established you as an indispensable witness to the unfolding narrative of this extraordinary journey.

The Bible reminds us that God never leaves us without a witness. I extend my heartfelt thanks to Brigette Levy and Yvonne O. Coke for their contributions and testimonies, serving as valuable witnesses in confirming the truth of this journey, just as the Bible emphasizes.[1] Your presence and support have been deeply appreciated.

---

1 2 Corinthians 13:1 (NIV)

To the dedicated team at TBN/Trilogy Publishing, who worked tirelessly to breathe life into this book and its stories of hope, I extend my deep gratitude. Your staunch dedication and boundless passion for this project made it a reality and elevated it to its fullest potential. Your collective effort and expertise have been instrumental in shaping this work and sharing its message with the world. Thank you for being invaluable partners on this transformative journey.

Finally, but certainly not least, I offer my gratitude to God for the precious gift of my son, Nathan, and for entrusting me with the profound responsibility of raising him and authentically sharing our story. It has been an immense privilege to serve as Nathan's mother and to facilitate his incredible potential and unique contributions to the world. I'm eagerly anticipating what the next phase of his life and our journey will gift us with.

Thank you all.

ENDORSEMENTS

Heart-wrenching and heartwarming simultaneously, Christine delivers with simplicity and charm. With thoughtful takeaways from challenging moments, it makes for a must-read for anyone who has a child with a disability.

—Anandita Oberoi, PhD, LPC
Adjunct Professor of Human Services
Editor of Human Services Today magazine,
National Organization for Human Services

Christine's authentic account of her journey in raising Nathan provides a roadmap that helps her audience understand the often hidden social, emotional, and physical challenges while also offering hope and actionable solutions for navigating the everyday life with a child with disabilities.

—Tara Malphrus-Sanchez
Special Education Teacher and Trainer

Christine, you have ignited the "warrior" spirit within us, demonstrating the power of unwavering advocacy for human rights. Your journey with Nathan is a rallying cry for families to recognize the strength they possess in the fight for recognition and support for their more vulnerable members. When my son (same age as Nathan) expressed his gratitude for the consistent support his father and I provided, I was reminded of the crucial battles you fought for your children and won. My son's acknowledgment of our refusal to be daunted by his challenges and our advocacy for him, especially in the educational setting, mirrored the unyielding determination of Christine when it came to Nathan.

Christine taught my family, friends, and me that our children's challenges are not a source of embarrassment but a call to action, a chance to stand against stigma and to secure their rightful place in society.

Your unyielding courage and fierce advocacy have empowered us to continue our journey with confidence and purpose. This book is not just an endorsement of Christine's efforts but a testament to the change she inspires in the lives she touches. Thank you for this book, championing the cause with such tenacity and reminding us that our fight can lead to significant strides in securing the rights of all and truly "leave no one behind."

—Curline Beckford,
Independent Consultant and Inclusive Advocate
(Fervently believing in a world where everyone has a rightful place and where there is recognition and protection of each individual's rights)

TABLE OF CONTENTS

Foreword..17

Reflection...21

Chapter 1—Unexpected News...29

Chapter 2—Let's Go Back to the Beginning of Our Story...........37

Chapter 3—When Life Changes in an Instant!............................49

Chapter 4—The Birth of This Gift from God.............................59

Chapter 5—Post-Delivery Realities..71

Chapter 6—Challenging Fate: Confronting the Odds 77

Chapter 7—The CDH Surgery...85

Chapter 8—Recovery and Hospital Stay 93

Chapter 9—Moments of Faith and Purpose..............................105

Chapter 10—Connecting Threads of Hope and Support.............113

Chapter 11—Through the Maze of Uncertainty:
              Our Journey to Diagnosis.....................................121

Chapter 12—The Road to Diagnosis:
              Fitting Together the Pieces of the Puzzle 129

Chapter 13—Understanding the Diagnosis:
              Moving Beyond Puzzle Pieces 135

Chapter 14—Acceptance's Long and Winding Road..................151

Chapter 15—The Day I Met My Son 161

Chapter 16—A Journey of Hope and Empowerment 171

Chapter 17—Awakening to Purpose...181

Chapter 18—The Power of Unconditional Acceptance...............191

Chapter 19—Journey Companions...............................199

Chapter 20—Trusting in God's Plan.............................207

Chapter 21—When the Pieces Fall in Place 221

Chapter 22—Same Story, Different Perspective:
            Robert's Account 231

Chapter 23—Same Story, Different Perspective:
            Adrianne's Account

Chapter 24—Ryan and Jordanne's Accounts...............................253

Chapter 25—Nathan's Account: This Gift from God 267

Chapter 26—Finding Harmony with God's Master Plan 281

Epilogue 297

About the Author..305

FOREWORD

As I write this foreword, I reflect on the compelling force of prayer, on what it means to be a partner in hope, and on the undeniable power of a mother's love.

A mother's love is a cradle to a child's soul and can never be fully estimated. And when you have a praying mother, her dedication, perseverance, relentless faith, and persistence in her child's purpose are unshakeable, unforgettable, and unapologetic. This love goes beyond measure because this mother stands with God in knowing that her child first belongs to Him, and no matter how difficult the journey, there are no mistakes for what God has created.

It is my joy to formally introduce a mother who embodies and bears this constitution. Her name is none other than Christine, which means follower of Christ. She is the mother of Nathan, Adrianne, Ryan, and Jordanne and the wife of Robert. Christine is also the author and light bearer of the book you hold in your hands.

I met Christine seventeen years ago, and we have been partners of hope ever since. In 2007, I arrived in Jamaica for the first time with my husband Russell to meet Christine and start a journey of aspiration and impact. We knew what we were in for, and despite the challenges ahead, we jointly signed up to change a school and then a nation! There are many stories to be told about our journey, but my heart firmly rests in the understanding that our meeting was destined and undoubtedly shepherded by God.

Take a few minutes and consider the most defining moments

of your life. Are their faces and feelings that are attached to your moments? How did those moments change you? Inspire you. Challenge you. How did the moments reveal more of who you are and the power of God? There have been a handful of experiences that have been completely life-altering for me. My journey with Christine is undoubtedly one of the most remarkable and unexpected!

There's something powerfully strange about traveling to a place you have never been before and letting go of familiar things to embrace something new. In situations like this, one may lean more softly or firmly into trusting God and having faith. In a tiny but meaningful way, I liken the power of Christine's journey in raising Nathan to this personal reflection. Embracing the unknown, trusting, and finding the glory of God even in the most uncertain times and the most unexpected and yet astonishing moments can be remarkably transformative.

I have firmly stood with Christine when her son, Nathan, was denied services, care, and support because of his diagnosis. Through my collaboration with her in Jamaica, I have witnessed fathers' sweat and tears after walking flights of stairs, carrying their ten-year-old and fourteen-year-old sons in their arms because there were no elevators or ramps for access in hopes of finding answers for care and service for their children. We have been ushered into homes where mothers cried to us that they want their children to be seen, known, felt, and recognized as human beings with rights. I have held Christine's hands in prayer, the same hands that have lifted her child and other people's children in prayer and with strength. At every turn of our journey, I see her advocacy, resilience, and profound commitment to widening the circle and perspective of God's grace for children and persons with disabilities.

Christine has a powerful discernment and courageously walks in faith and conviction by sharing her story. I feel blessed to witness her love for her son, her family, and the advocacy of families whose voices have been silenced or suppressed. Christine is a model of inspiration, and by telling her story, she influences other parents to find the courage to share their stories too.

As our dear friend Sidney Morrison once wrote: We are the stories we tell. We are the stories we tell about ourselves and others. They define us; they inspire, provoke, explain, nurture, and console us.

The experience of faith and parenting are powerful, and both actions come with a story; whether you're a parent by birth, by love, or by a child's nomination, we often find ourselves being the advocates for our children's wellness, sense of belonging, their God-given rights, and protections.

Through her words and lived experience, Christine invites us to take her hand, tear down the fences of separation, and walk intimately into the privacies of her heart as she reveals her parenting journey with her son, Nathan, and with God. This journey is intimate, captivating, compelling, and necessary in understanding and raising a child to thrive with disabilities. Christine acknowledges her pain and the spiritual and psychological wounds of mothering a child with special needs, and she brings forth her triumphs and the redemptive nature of God's promise. She makes her wisdom, truth, challenges, and love accessible to us all through examples of soul-comforting moments and earthly stories with heavenly meanings.

This book is a much-needed gift to all of us. May Christine's words inspire you, transform you, and remind you of King David's proclamation of one of God's most extraordinary plans, "For you created my inmost being; you knit me together in my mother's womb. I praise you because I am fearfully and wonderfully made" (Psalm 139:13–14).

Let us glorify God and wholeheartedly dare to see all children as image bearers of His beauty, wholeness, and greatness.

Your sister, by and in Spirit,

—Senta Greene, MA, CCLS,
a leading expert in reimagining education and inclusion for children's social justice.

REFLECTION

When I penned and published my very first book, *Raising Nathan: Every Life Has a Story*,[2] Nathan was just ten years old. At that time, I was still wrestling with the weight of my own journey, struggling to make sense of my pain, and feeling like I lacked so much, including the support I desperately sought. As a result, the story I shared in that book reflected my raw and unfiltered experiences.

My primary focus then revolved around the challenges we faced and the darker aspects of our journey. I fixated on what we had lost, our shattered dreams, unfulfilled aspirations, and the ever-present uncertainty that cast a shadow over our futures. I found it incredibly difficult to identify any lessons, distill meaningful messages, or detect a trace of hope within our situation.

There was no one I could turn to for help with what I was going through, mainly because it wasn't the norm in my Jamaican culture. You see, living in Jamaica, seeking counseling or professional help was not something that people typically did. Mental health wasn't discussed much during those times, and we were raised believing that family problems should stay within the family and that we shouldn't share our issues with the outside world. So, concealing my struggles within became my automatic reaction.

To compound an already challenging situation, the stigma surrounding disability persisted strongly and was deeply in-

---

2 Christine Staple Ebanks, Raising Nathan: Every Life Has a Story (Kingston, Jamaica: Nathan Ebanks Foundation, 2015).

grained in our culture. Children with disabilities often were in-visible, hidden, or even abandoned. I vividly recall growing up alongside neighbors who would bring a new baby home, only for that child to mysteriously vanish from our sight, never to be seen again. Years later, after my son's diagnosis, some of these people confessed that their child had a disability and were either kept inside, given up to the children's home, or sent to live with distant relatives in rural areas.

In one particularly heart-wrenching case, a family put their eight-year-old son with autism to bed and immigrated to En-gland, leaving in the middle of the night while he slept. When I finally had the opportunity to meet him, he was fifty-five years old, and his response when asked about his family was, "Family gone. I woke up, and they had left me."

Our society provided little to no education or awareness about this particular group of people. In fact, during my childhood, I was taught not to make eye contact with individuals who were blind, had mobility issues, or had visible physical disabilities. As a result, we naturally severed the human connection with those who appeared different from us, rendering them invisible within our communities.

So, when we received Nathan's diagnosis of cerebral palsy against this backdrop, I felt the weight of our culture pressing down on me. Burdened by shame, guilt, and fear, it seemed as if our world had plunged into an abyss of despair. Additionally, I carried the burden of fearing that I lacked the knowledge and abilities to be his best mother. The worry that I might fall short of my duty to provide proper care and the concern that the world would never fully accept him was a heavy load to bear. Further-more, I was apprehensive that my friends would perceive me differently; sadly, some did.

I vividly remember a time when our financial situation became particularly challenging. In Jamaica, the full cost of caring for a child with a disability falls upon the immediate family, primarily the parents. By the time Nathan started kindergarten, our family was facing financial difficulties due to the cost for him and his three siblings in elementary school. I was grappling with the challenge of maintaining our household. During this tough period, I unexpectedly met someone who happened to know one of my older sisters at a popular park one day. Later, I discovered from my sister that this individual had shared their embarrassment regarding my appearance. In their words, I appeared to be "suffering," a term reminiscent of colonial times that conveys financial hardship or destitution. They recommended that my sister counsel me to dress appropriately before going out in public.

That was my rock-bottom moment. It was the time when I humbly surrendered everything about my life at God's feet. I gently reminded Him (although I knew He needed no reminder) that He gave me this "gift" of my son and his diagnosis and that my family and I serve as His witnesses and a living expression of His testimony on earth. In answer to my prayer, God conveyed a clear message through various individuals, some of whom I was acquainted with, while others were complete strangers. They all urged me to write, telling me that there was redemption, hope, and healing within my story. Their words echoed with a resounding message that there are people waiting for my perspective. It didn't make sense to me and didn't magically solve my problems. However, I decided to heed their counsel and take action. In obedience to that calling, I embarked on the journey of writing and self-publishing my very first book on raising Nathan.

My story flowed with raw emotions in that initial book, and my pain and struggles were palpable. I couldn't help but wonder if anyone would genuinely be interested in what I had to share. After all, there were numerous books authored by subject matter experts and parents who had walked similar paths with their children with disabilities. I had purchased and read several of those books myself. However, deep down, I carried the awareness that certain essential aspects of my experience remained unaddressed in the books I had heard and read. These books primarily delved into medical, special education services, social services, and disability laws, some of which did not reflect my specific context.

Furthermore, some of these resources took a purely spiritual approach, lacking the practical application I desperately needed. My frustration deepened because I was aware that I didn't understand my son's diagnosis or how to help him. I also understood that, without the necessary guidance, I was in a situation where I didn't even know what I didn't know.

Then, something truly remarkable occurred. About a year after I released that initial book, people started sharing how it had profoundly blessed their lives. One vivid memory stands out when I traveled through the airport in Jamaica on my way to an event in San Francisco in 2016. I was pulled out of the line as I passed the departure security checkpoint. The customs officer approached me, reassuring me that my bags were in order. However, her true motive was to meet me because she had recognized that I was the author of *Raising Nathan*. She went on to explain that several weeks before, an outgoing passenger had inadvertently left their copy of my book, along with an expensive pen, in the airport lounge. Her supervisor had discovered the book and started reading it, unable to tear herself away from its pages.

She continued, oblivious to the people who were waiting in line behind me to pass through the checkpoint. She said, "Miss, I don't typically enjoy reading. But from the moment I started reading your book, I couldn't put it down. I laughed, cried, prayed, got angry, and journeyed with you through the story. I celebrated the wins, clapping my hands in joy, often startling my children, for it was as if I was right there beside you. I don't have a child with a disability, but I have young children. Your book taught me how important it is to listen to and speak up for my children. It also showed me the importance of speaking up for children with disabilities in my community and giving these mothers an encouraging word when I see them. Thank you for writing this book and sharing your story; it has not only changed my perspective but also transformed my life."

As she spoke, I felt my cheeks flush with embarrassment. I didn't know how to respond except to say, "Thank you." After all, I had written the book as a means of personal expression and in obedience to God, without any other specific goals in mind. As I walked away, I noticed other passengers who had been eavesdropping on our conversation, smiling at me. It dawned on me that the scanner picked up the book when my bag was inspected.

This airport encounter marked the first of many similar instances where individuals who read my book or heard me speak reached out to share how my story had deeply touched their lives. It left me puzzled for a while because I still couldn't fully see the true extent of the story's power.

Then, a few years later, I spoke at a New York fundraiser. It was purely by chance for one man in the audience. He had never heard of me and had only come along because he was giving a friend a ride to the event. As fate would have it, he walked in just as I took the stage, and my story grabbed hold of him in an unexpected way.

Afterward, he approached me, eager to share his own moving story. He explained that while he didn't know anyone with a disability, he was battling a significant issue in his life that had left him teetering on the brink of giving up. However, listening to my story touched him deeply, soul-stirringly. It made him realize that our pain and struggles aren't meant to break us; they can guide us toward a more purposeful path. He felt as though I had spoken directly about his own situation, and he wanted to express his gratitude for my vulnerability and my ability to see my son's challenge as an opportunity to find solutions for him and others. With a smile, he shared that I had helped him change the lens through which he had been viewing his own situation.

This feedback marked yet another defining moment. I realized it wasn't about my perceptions but how God chose to use my life and my son's. It reaffirmed that even in this situation, God had a purpose for my life and used Nathan as an integral part of His unfolding plan. At that very moment, I made a resolute decision to be His willing vessel.

The book you are currently holding originally began as an update to the original work, *Raising Nathan: Every Life Has a Story*. In 2020, my family and I immigrated to the United States, and Nathan's life underwent significant changes and growth. In 2023, as Nathan turned eighteen, updating the book became an imperative, representing the logical and seamless next step. However, a mere two months into the writing process, a major health event involving Nathan unfolded, leading to a profound shift from updating the book to the inception of an entirely new project. This endeavor entailed a comprehensive reimagining of the early facets of the story, incorporating fresh accounts and experiences spanning the years leading up to his current age.

This broader approach provides a more comprehensive perspective on the extraordinary journey of raising Nathan against formidable odds from birth to adulthood. Furthermore, this longitudinal view makes the profound presence of God's grace, provision, and numerous other blessings more evident.

In addition, I have attempted to relay key defining moments that strengthened my faith, giving me practical glimpses of God in the "everythingness" of life. Equally, it is about how, in brokenness, God uses the journey of raising my son to unlock precious gifts—expressed in faith, blessings, joy, family, community, resilience, and purpose. He has shown me how all of these experiences were catalysts to draw out transformation and help me evolve into a better version of myself.

My sole request as you read this book is to open your hearts and minds, allowing the spirit of God to connect with you wherever you may be on your journey. As I've realized, greatness resides within each of us, irrespective of our abilities or disabilities. We are all created in the image and likeness of God, each with a unique purpose. Whether we are parents, professionals, believers, or members of civil society, we all have a role to fulfill and something valuable to offer in this journey called life. With this in mind, I humbly present *Raising Nathan Against All Odds: Discovering the Blessings, Joy, and Purpose in Raising a Child with Disabilities.*

CHAPTER 1

UNEXPECTED NEWS

A Moment Frozen in Time

As I stood in the hospital's emergency room, my mind was filled with a mixture of fear and uncertainty. Once again, my youngest son, Nathan, was fighting for his life. The doctors' explanations echoed in my ears, their serious tone and concerned expressions revealing the gravity of his situation. It was evident that Nathan's condition was serious.

Just the day before, my third-born, Jordanne, and I had taken Nathan to the mall to indulge in two of his favorite activities—people-watching and savoring delicious food. Jordanne, who was home from graduate school where she studies speech and language pathology, thought it would be a wonderful way for Nathan to enjoy the pre-Easter festivities. We watched as he had an amazing time, even posing for pictures with the Easter Bunny at a delightful pop-up photo booth.

However, when Nathan started throwing up that night, my first thought was that he might have consumed something disagreeable at the mall. Throughout the night, his condition persisted, prompting me to take precautionary measures. Following my usual practice, I scheduled a telehealth visit with a doctor from his pediatrician clinic to seek guidance.

During the virtual visit, the doctor acknowledged my suspicion that Nathan might have caught a bug, as she had been observing similar symptoms in many of her young patients. She prescribed an anti-nausea medication and advised me to ensure his hydration. Due to Nathan's cerebral palsy, she recommended that taking him to the emergency room (ER) would be prudent if his condition persisted over the next two days.

The next day was Good Friday, and his condition had worsened. Every ounce of fluids he took in came back shortly after—the force of his vomit was unlike anything I had ever seen. Nathan, who always wears a cheerful disposition and a disarming smile, was now restless, squirming in pain, and grimacing. Because he is nonverbal, he couldn't tell me his feelings. I attempted to use his communication device to understand what he was experiencing and where he was experiencing pain. But his distress was so great that our usual method of communication proved ineffective. This heightened my worry, as I had never witnessed him in such distressing circumstances.

Since Robert had just gone to bed after his all-night job, I talked with Ryan, my second-born, who was awake. I expressed my worries about Nathan's worsening condition, and he agreed that something wasn't right with Nathan. We both felt that to be on the safe side, we should take him to the ER right away. Before I could ask for help, Ryan offered to come along, and I was grateful for this support.

As I stepped through the doors of the ER that Friday morning, a familiar mix of anxiety, trepidation, and fear settled in the pit of my stomach. It was a sensation I had grown accustomed to since the day Nathan was born. However, I consciously pushed those thoughts aside, reassuring myself that this was likely just a stomach bug. I held onto the hope that Nathan would receive the necessary hydration and, if needed, antibiotics for a potential infection. In my mind, we would be in and out of the hospital, returning home by the end of the day.

Nathan was swiftly attended to in the triage area, and within thirty minutes, he was settled in a bed in the ER, receiving much-needed hydration fluids. His restlessness had escalated significantly, and he intermittently cried out in distress. It was unsettling, not just for me but also for Ryan, who had never witnessed such behavior from Nathan before. His constant squirming and writhing posed challenges for the nurses as they worked to secure the intravenous lines (IV lines)[3]. I deeply appreciated their patience and expertise throughout the process.

While the nurses worked with him, one of them engaged me in conversation, asking questions to gather his medical history from when I was pregnant to his birth, diagnosis, and other significant health events. This served as a welcome distraction from the distressing scene unfolding before me. Recounting his history is a familiar litany for me, as I have shared the stories and chronology of events numerous times over the years. The details had become ingrained in my memory, a testament to the journey we had traversed together and the numerous obstacles we had surmounted.

The room buzzed with activity as various medical practitioners

---

3 IV lines are used to deliver fluids, medications, or nutrients directly into the bloodstream. IV lines are commonly used in medical settings to provide various treatments and interventions.

entered and exited, each focused on their specific tasks. With every procedure performed, the teams took the time to explain to me what they were doing. The range of tests felt overwhelming, from X-rays to CT scans with contrast and comprehensive blood profiles. However, amidst the whirlwind of activity, I found reassurance in witnessing the diligence of the medical team. Evidently, they were working assiduously to identify the underlying problem and provide the necessary care for Nathan.

After a while, a doctor entered the room accompanied by a small team, identifying himself as the head of the Colon and Rectal Surgery department. In that moment, it felt as if time stood still, and I was transported back to the vivid memories of that fateful day eighteen years ago. It was the day I learned that Nathan had been diagnosed with congenital diaphragmatic hernia (CDH), a life-threatening condition that necessitated immediate and complex surgical intervention. The only difference was that back then, Nathan was still in the womb, and I was merely five months pregnant, facing a terrifying unknown.

I shook myself out of the memories, consciously grounding myself in the present moment. The distressing reality was undeniable: something was seriously wrong with Nathan's health. As I whispered a prayer for strength, calmness, and peace, I braced myself for the news that the doctors were about to deliver.

DIAGNOSIS: INTESTINAL OBSTRUCTION

With my heart pounding, I anxiously waited for the doctor to speak. Ryan stood quietly beside me, his hand resting gently on my shoulder, offering a reassuring squeeze that reminded me I was not alone. In that moment, I couldn't help but recognize the eerie familiarity of fear and uncertainty that enveloped me. It felt as though these emotions were familiar companions, faithfully reemerging over the years whenever a crisis concerning Nathan loomed.

"Mrs. Ebanks, as you know, we conducted a series of tests to investigate the underlying cause of Nathan's persistent vomiting. We have identified a blockage in Nathan's intestines based on the results of the X-rays and CT scan with contrast. It appears that there may be some accumulation of old stool causing the obstruction, but it could also indicate a more significant issue. Our current plan is to keep Nathan overnight, administer an enema to attempt to alleviate the blockage, and reassess his condition in the morning. If the obstruction does not resolve with these measures, immediate surgery will be necessary."

A familiar ache settled within my heart as the doctor's words sank in. I released a slow exhale, feeling the weight of the uncertainties and the countless ifs that filled the air. I turned my gaze toward Nathan, his fragile form lying in the hospital bed. Despite his drowsiness and a slightly calmer disposition than when we first arrived, it was evident that he was still in pain. My heart shattered for him, and in that moment, I longed to trade places with him, to bear the burden on his behalf. It felt deeply unjust that at such a young age, he had already endured more hardships than many would encounter in their entire lives.

The weight of the situation settled upon my shoulders, and the realization that I was once again being called to be "his voice" was overwhelming and exhausting. Tiredness washed over me as my inner self screamed, *Oh no, not again. I don't know if I can go through this once more.* But, amidst the fatigue, my logical voice steadfastly reminded me of my responsibility to ensure Nathan received the best care and support, ensuring he never felt alone during this health crisis.

As I was lost in my thoughts, my mind raced with the logistics of what needed to be done. It became evident that we required a well-structured schedule to ensure someone was constantly by Nathan's side in the hospital, providing him with the round-the-clock support he was accustomed to receiving. Maintaining this sense of normalcy was crucial for him, especially as he was used to having one of us present whenever he wasn't at school. However, I couldn't help but wonder how we would manage it all, considering that Robert, Adrianne (our oldest), and Ryan had their work commitments.

Just as these concerns consumed me, I felt a gentle touch on the small of my back and turned to see Adrianne standing behind me. Ryan had stepped out to make a call and update our family at home, and he had reached out to Adrianne, who had immediately left work to join us at the hospital. Despite being only eight years older than Nathan, Adrianne had always assumed a maternal role with him, affectionately referring to him as "her baby." Her presence was reassuring.

Shortly after, I received a call from Robert informing me that he had taken the night off from work and was on his way to the hospital to stay with Nathan throughout the night. He insisted that I go home and get some much-needed rest. By the time Robert arrived, it was already past eight in the evening, and I had spent over eight hours at the hospital. With no immediate decisions to be made until the morning, I reluctantly agreed to take his advice and headed home.

We left the hospital (Ryan, Adrianne, and me) shortly after Robert arrived. As we walked to the parking lot, Adrianne leaned over and embraced me tightly. She whispered in my ear, "Mom, I finally understand what you and Daddy went through when Nathan was in the hospital after he was born. I can't imagine how you both managed it. Ryan, Jordanne, and I were still so young back then, and we couldn't offer much help. As I stand here now, my heart breaks for Natey Bear. I want to thank you for everything you did for him and for our family. I want you to know that you and Daddy are not alone this time. We are here, and we will help carry the load."

Adrianne's words touched me deeply. I couldn't help but feel gratitude for her and her siblings' care, concern, and support that day. While I have always known their deep love for their little brother, witnessing it on display filled my heart with immense joy and relief. It was then that I knew this time things would be different. Unlike when Nathan was born, we now had the physical and emotional help of our older children to navigate whatever lay ahead.

Ryan insisted on taking the wheel for the journey back home, and I was grateful. Thankfully, our home was just a short ten-minute drive away. As we traveled along the familiar route, I could feel the weight of exhaustion descending upon me. However, this time, it felt different. Instead of dread and despair, there was gratitude and hope. Though I did not yet know what challenges were ahead, there was a quiet reassurance that all was well.

When we arrived home, I got a quick bite to eat before taking a shower and going to bed. I fell asleep almost immediately.

TAKEAWAY

Throughout my journey of raising Nathan, I've encountered unexpected news repeatedly. It's become clear to me that fear and uncertainty are natural human reactions when faced with such news. Recognizing and accepting these emotions as a normal part of the journey has enabled me to develop emotional resilience and approach challenges with greater strength.

Another vital lesson that has deeply shaped my point of view is the pivotal role of my faith in guiding me through the multitude of challenges we've encountered over the years. This transformation didn't occur overnight but rather unfolded gradually through a series of diverse experiences. Confronting circumstances that often lay beyond our control, particularly those involving my child, has been a source of significant spiritual enrichment, fostering a strong and steadfast connection with my faith.

CHAPTER 2

LET'S GO BACK TO THE BEGINNING OF OUR STORY

Life Interrupted

The unexpected news of Nathan's arrival took us completely by surprise. My husband, Robert, and I were happily married for seven years and raising three young children. While his arrival was not part of our plans, in hindsight, subtle signs hinted at his impending arrival about a year before.

The chain of events began during a serene moment at church while I was fully engrossed in the Good Friday morning sermon. Out of nowhere, I was overwhelmed by a vivid vision of myself, heavily pregnant. The experience was so incredibly lifelike that I felt compelled to share it with my sister, Jennifer, as soon as I returned home after the service. To my annoyance, she found it utterly amusing and jokingly remarked, "Chris, you would definitely die if you were to get pregnant now!" I couldn't help but nod in agreement, recognizing the truth in her jest.

At that time, my life felt perfectly imbalanced-balanced. Robert and I were excelling in our respective careers—he in finance, and I in marketing. We already had our hands full with our busy schedules and the responsibilities of raising a young family. Therefore, adding another baby seemed completely out of the question. It simply wasn't part of our plans, and we felt content with how things were.

As time went by, the vision gradually receded into the background of my mind. I settled into a comfortable rhythm in life, embracing my daily routine. However, a little over a year later, everything changed. One morning, I woke up feeling unusually off. My body was exhausted as if I had just completed a grueling marathon the previous day. Despite the overwhelming fatigue, I pushed myself to head out to work, knowing I had an important corporate event to organize and a series of back-to-back meetings.

I arrived at work later than usual but found concentrating increasingly challenging. As the day progressed, my condition continued to deteriorate. Eventually, after a few hours of struggling, I realized that it would be in my best interest to return home.

Just as I reached for the phone to call my shared assistant, Rose-Marie, to ask for her help to reschedule my meetings, I heard a voice say, "You are pregnant!" Startled, I turned around, but there was no one but me in my semi-enclosed office. I picked up the phone, and as I dialed Rose-Marie's number, I heard the same voice repeat, "You are pregnant!"

Feeling apprehensive, I decided to go to Rose-Marie's desk to talk to her. However, as I stood up, an intense prickling sensation surged through my body, shooting to my feet and toes. Alarmed by this unexpected numbing feeling, I quickly sat back down. Rose-Marie walked in at that moment and, seeing the look on my face, asked if I was feeling okay. I confessed that I wasn't and shared how I was feeling. She agreed that I should head home and that she would reschedule my meetings.

As I gathered my belongings, a fleeting thought crossed my mind once more: I was pregnant again. But I swiftly brushed it aside, deeming it too far-fetched. However, despite my attempts to push it away, the feeling persisted, growing more insistent with each passing moment. Unable to ignore this nagging feeling, I decided to stop at a pharmacy to purchase a pregnancy kit on my way home. I rationalized that this would help me get peace of mind and some much-needed rest once I ruled out the possibility of being pregnant.

Just as I was about to leave my office, the phone ringing interrupted my thoughts. It was Karyn, one of the contractors for the event, calling because Rose-Marie had yet to be successful in contacting her. She wanted me to know she was running late for our meeting but was on her way. I explained the situation and that Rose-Marie would call her to reschedule. However, before we concluded the call, she requested a small favor from me. Despite a twinge of regret that surfaced upon hearing Karyn's request, I didn't hesitate to agree. She wanted me to collect an envelope from another department, with the plan to meet up later to retrieve it from me.

As fate would have it, the pharmacy I intended to visit happened to be the perfect rendezvous point. A brief moment of hesitation gripped me, as I did not want to reveal the true reason for my visit to the pharmacy. However, a glimmer of a plan formed in my mind—I could arrive at the pharmacy before Karyn, swiftly make my purchase, and then meet her in the parking lot. This way, I could maintain my privacy while still fulfilling the favor. The idea seemed sound, offering me a semblance of control over the situation. I resolved to hand Karyn the envelope discreetly in the parking lot, keeping the possibility of pregnancy concealed.

As I pulled into the pharmacy's parking lot, a sinking feeling washed over me when I caught sight of Karyn's car already parked there. My worries intensified, but I gathered my composure and parked my car beside hers. Putting on a smile, I handed her the envelope, hoping to conclude the interaction swiftly. However, to my dismay, Karyn seemed eager to engage in conversation and showed no signs of leaving. I discreetly glanced at my watch, silently urging her to pick up on my cues to go. Yet, she remained oblivious to my subtle hints.

Spurred on by the urgency of my goal to purchase the pregnancy kit in secret, I wrapped up the conversation and said goodbye. I turned toward the pharmacy, but my heart sank when she exclaimed that she was heading there. I didn't want to be rude, so I continued walking. But to my relief, she turned toward the entrance of the adjacent supermarket instead. Sighing with relief, I entered the pharmacy alone, finally able to address my purpose without the prying eyes of others.

With a mixture of anticipation and anxiety, I made my choice and proceeded toward the checkout line. Yet, as I reached into my handbag to retrieve my purse, I could see it clearly in my mind's eye—resting on the kitchen counter at home, where I had put it that morning after giving my children their lunch money.

I rummaged through my handbag, hoping to find cash, but was unsuccessful. However, just as I turned to leave, a familiar voice reached my ears—it was Karyn standing behind me, offering to pay for the item. I had failed to notice her arrival in the pharmacy, but she must have caught sight of my predicament and stepped forward to help. Caught off guard, I found myself momentarily speechless, unable to respond. Before I could gather my thoughts, she swiftly paid the cashier, collected the item, and handed it to me with a warm smile.

Overwhelmed by the unexpected turn of events, I was at a loss for words. Embarrassment washed over me, reminiscent of a child caught with their hand in the cookie jar. Offering a hasty thank-you, I retreated, hoping to escape the situation. Yet, to my distress, Karyn followed me, seemingly oblivious to my discomfort. She asked if I thought I might be pregnant.

Caught off balance, I struggled to find a response, leaving an awkward silence between us. Sensing my unease, it was then that she realized she had overstepped her boundaries and promptly apologized. However, on the back of the apology, she started talking about her own struggles with infertility with her new husband. Despite having raised children from a previous marriage, she had difficulties conceiving again. She said she felt that her infertility could mean the end of her marriage. While I empathized deeply with her pain, my own predicament consumed my thoughts. So, I said nothing. After a brief pause, Karyn bid me farewell. As she walked away, her words floated back, "I hope you are pregnant. If you are, enjoy the gift."

THE MOMENT OF TRUTH

I sat alone in my car in the parking lot, enveloped in a heavy silence. Suddenly, the urgency to know if I was pregnant became unbearable—I couldn't bear to wait until I reached home. I dialed the numbers of my brother Michael and sister Jennifer, who both lived nearby. I decided to go to my brother's home since he was home, and Jennifer was still at work.

I arrived at Michael's home quickly, and after greeting him, I asked him to use his bathroom. He looked at me curiously. Entering the bathroom, I closed the door and leaned against it. Now that the moment of truth had arrived, I wasn't sure I wanted to go through with it. It took me a moment to gather my courage, and then I took the test. But I felt certain I was pregnant even before I saw the confirmation: two vibrant pink lines with the word "positive."

Nonetheless, the confirmation rocked me off my feet. I sat down hard on the toilet seat as a deluge of emotions washed over me—fear, apprehension, disbelief, with a touch of excitement. I was confused. Then panic rushed in as I thought about what a new pregnancy may mean. My body had barely recovered from my pregnancy with Jordanne three years before, and the idea of doing it all over again seemed daunting. I had no idea how I was going to manage it all.

Realizing I couldn't stay in my brother's bathroom forever, I washed my hands and face and walked into the living room. Michael was standing there looking worried. He asked if I was okay, and I managed to answer with a smile. Finally, I blurted out, "I'm pregnant." But, to my surprise and annoyance, he chuckled and then laughed outright, his booming laughter bouncing off the living room walls. I was annoyed. "I'm glad you find humor in this," I snapped at him. "No, it's not that," he replied. "I would have told you not to take a pregnancy test in *that* bathroom if I knew you would do that. No pregnancy test has ever been taken there that came back negative." I saw the irony since he and his wife had two pregnancies in quick succession.

Despite my brother's attempt to lighten the mood, I couldn't find the humor in the situation. Confirming my pregnancy brought other issues to the forefront of my thoughts. After saying goodbye, I left my brother's place and merged onto the main road, only to find myself stuck in the height of Friday evening traffic. My travel time home had now become considerably longer than earlier in the day. However, I found gratitude in this delay, as it provided me with the time I needed to organize my thoughts and prepare for breaking the news to Robert.

THIS GIFT FROM GOD

As I was stuck behind a long line of traffic, my mind couldn't escape the pressing concern of how to tell Robert we were pregnant—again. It had only been a matter of weeks since we joyfully celebrated the potty-training achievement of our young daughter, Jordanne. So, how could another baby be on the way already? Having had three children in five years had left us sleep-deprived and stretched thin from midnight feedings, financial, and other

43

countless responsibilities of raising young children. In addition, Robert was on the cusp of completing his master's degree, which meant he could finally reclaim his evenings after years of juggling midnight feedings, early morning wake-ups, and studying on top of his job.

As I crawled along with the traffic, my mind was consumed with worry about how Robert would react to the unexpected pregnancy news. I was going through the driving motions almost on autopilot; my thoughts were elsewhere as I navigated the busy streets. Despite my attempts to focus on the road, my mind kept returning to the fear and uncertainty that had taken hold. Though I knew deep down that he would be supportive and loving, I couldn't shake off the fear that he might not take the news well, especially since I wasn't taking it well either.

It was dark when I finally pulled into our driveway. I turned off the engine but sat in my car, trying to find the courage to go in and tell Robert the news. In the stillness of the evening, the situation loomed larger than life. Consumed by thoughts of the countless ways a new baby would change my life—physically, mentally, and emotionally—I was instantly overcome by a wave of overwhelming emotions. Memories flooded back, recounting the physical changes my body would undergo, the demands of pregnancy, childbirth, and night feedings. Contemplating these aspects left me utterly drained, and I wrestled with the question of where I would find the strength to do it all over again.

On the other hand, Robert is an amazing father and an incredibly loving and supportive husband who goes above and beyond to ensure my and our children's comfort. I still remember when

I was pregnant with Jordanne, how he once drove for hours in the middle of the night to get me pickles so that I could settle a pregnancy craving. However, as I thought about what was to come, another concern gnawed at my heart. It had been difficult for us to keep pace with the demands of our current little ones. The sleepless nights, endless responsibilities, and the relentless juggling act had taken their toll on our marriage. Now, confronted with the reality of a new baby, I wondered how it would impact the delicate balance we had managed to establish. *Would our relationship withstand the strain? Would we find the strength to navigate this new chapter together, or would it further stretch the limits of our endurance?* The thought of adding more stress to an already strained dynamic filled me with apprehension and uncertainty. I just didn't know how to break the news to him.

As I sat behind the wheel of my car, feeling overwhelmed and in need of guidance, I reached out to God through prayer, asking for wisdom and direction. Then, unexpectedly, the same gentle voice that had spoken to me earlier in the day broke through the silence, "Tell Robert that this child is a gift from God. With this child, you will prove Me (God)." Stunned by the message, I wondered if it was an answer from God or merely a creation of my own imagination. However, the words resonated with a resounding conviction, cutting through the doubts and uncertainties that had clouded my mind moments before. I felt the first seed of hope since discovering my pregnancy. I felt at peace. It was time to tell Robert.

Filled with renewed energy from this profound spiritual encounter, I exited the car and walked up the short flight of steps to the front door. I stepped into the living room, where Robert was deeply engrossed in his studies, seated comfortably on the couch. As my presence interrupted his concentration, he looked up, his face breaking into a warm and affectionate smile. Our eyes locked, and in that fleeting moment, I basked in the familiar, comforting warmth in his eyes that always made me feel adored and cherished. However, his lingering gaze also carried an air of expectation this time. It was as if he sensed that I had something important to share.

As I gathered the courage to speak, the words "We're pregnant" escaped my lips. However, to my surprise, Robert's reaction was not shock or dismay. It was as though he had already intuited the news. He smiled reassuringly. "This is great news!" he exclaimed. "I can't wait to see the look of excitement on the children's faces when we tell them they will have a new brother or sister."

Instantly, the weight I had been carrying lifted, replaced by peace and a flickering of excitement. We spoke for a while about what it would mean in the physical space for us to have this new baby. We mused about the "gift" this child would bring. Maybe he or she will be a great athlete. A talented musician or a great evangelist. As we spoke, I thought about the greats in the Bible: Moses, Sampson, David, Elijah, Esther, and Deborah. My heart filled with hope with each thought.

As I lay in bed later that night, I felt a sense of hope and wonder in my heart. One cannot equate the joy and love of having a new baby with that newborn baby smell, witnessing their milestones, and experiencing their unconditional love. In addition, I had long believed that life is sacred and that children are God's blessings. The assurance that this child is a gift from God filled me with exhilarating anticipation. It ignited boundless possibilities for him or her.

TAKEAWAY

The key takeaway from this chapter is that life often surprises us when we least expect it. In my life, this unexpected twist took the form of an unplanned pregnancy, which initially seemed like a disruption, a departure from the path I had carefully planned for myself. However, I soon came to realize there was a divine plan at play, a purpose beyond my immediate understanding. This unexpected twist in my life turned out to be a great blessing that would unfold in the ensuing years. It reinforced the notion that life's most exquisite moments often arise from the most unexpected circumstances, highlighting that sometimes the most wonderful things occur when we are least prepared for them.

CHAPTER 3

WHEN LIFE CHANGES IN AN INSTANT!

After coming to terms with the pregnancy, we were excited to share the news with our family. At six weeks, we gathered our parents and siblings to reveal the joyous secret. We told our children at three months, when inquisitive as ever, they kept asking why Mommy was getting fatter. We had chosen not to tell them too early, knowing their concept of time was still developing, and we wanted to spare them (and ourselves) the constant anticipation of the baby's arrival. Little did we know that they would soon take it upon themselves to spread the news far and wide, proudly announcing to strangers in the supermarket or even at Sunday service, "We are having a baby, and that's why Mommy is getting fat."

However, as the days passed, they would ask, "Is the baby coming today?" I would explain that the baby was still growing and needed to stay inside to become strong. To help them better grasp the concept of pregnancy, we bought a delightful 3D children's book about the developing fetus. It quickly became their favorite, and they would spend countless hours absorbed in its pages, talking together about the different stages of development.

Seeing their eagerness after school, racing to grab the book and discover the next chapter of the baby's growth, was delightful. Whenever we had visitors, they proudly proclaimed our impending arrival, enthusiastically sharing their newfound knowledge from the book. We couldn't help but smile at their infectious excitement and "expert" opinions. Witnessing their deep investment in the pregnancy was a remarkable foreshadowing of what lay ahead—the extraordinary power and beauty of sibling love. Little did we know then that this bond would prove invaluable in the years that followed.

While we were thrilled about our newest family member's arrival, the pregnancy proved challenging. From the very beginning, I experienced intense morning sickness and discomfort. To help take my mind off the discomfort, we started a friendly naming competition between the boys and girls in our family. The girls hoped for another girl, while the boys wished for a little boy. Ryan, who was six years old, believed it was only fair for us to have another boy, given that the girls in our family outnumbered the boys three to two. Despite the ongoing debate, though we didn't yet know the baby's sex, we curiously settled on two names, Jonathan and Nathan, both meaning "gift of God."

However, our lives took an unexpected turn during a routine prenatal visit at the five-month mark.

AN UNEXPECTED CHALLENGE

It was an ordinary Friday, December 12, 2003, when an unexpected shift occurred during our routine prenatal visit. Robert decided to accompany me that day, deviating from our usual routine, where I attended the visits alone after the initial appointment. Our conversations in the doctor's office were always lively and cheerful. Dr. Sideman looked forward to my visits, knowing that I would regale him with amusing anecdotes about my pregnancy-induced quirks and developments.

During the examination, I jokingly complained about my vanishing waistline and the newfound struggle of rolling out of bed in the mornings. I shared an incident where a business meeting ran late, cutting into my usual baby-fixed eating time, bringing me to the brink of tears. Dr. Sideman's laughter filled the small examination room as he proceeded with the ultrasound test. However, as he was about to leave the room to let me get dressed, he suddenly realized that he still needed to print the scan result. He quickly returned to continue scanning my belly, and everything changed at that moment. The once lighthearted atmosphere in the room abruptly shifted toward somberness, leaving me bewildered and concerned.

Dr. Sideman's laughter abruptly faded, leaving behind a disconcerting silence that hung in the air. I watched as his perplexed expression deepened, intensifying the moment's gravity. With each movement of the probe over my pregnant belly, he whispered, "This can't be right... How could I have missed this?" Icy fingers of fear crept from the depths of my core, gripping my heart and causing it to sink as I wondered what it was that he missed. I had never encountered such a disquieting situation throughout my previous three pregnancies. The sense of unease grew stronger, amplifying the intensity of the moment.

Despite my best efforts to remain composed, my stomach

tightened with a sense of dread. So caught up I was in the moment I forgot about Robert, who stood quietly by my side. I was struck by how swiftly the atmosphere in the room had shifted from laughter to an oppressive heaviness casting its somber shadow. I was desperate for Dr. Sideman to tell me what had him so concerned yet simultaneously apprehensive about what he might unveil.

After a while, I asked, "What did you miss, doctor? Is there something wrong with my baby?" While I anxiously waited for him to break the excruciating silence with any words, an inexplicable feeling washed over me as if our lives were on the cusp of yet another significant shift. I couldn't pinpoint how or through what means, but I had an overwhelming sense that something momentous was approaching. I longed to understand, yet a part of me resisted because I understood that everything would be forever changed the moment I knew.

After what seemed like an interminable wait, Dr. Sideman finally told me to get dressed and exited the room. My heart raced as I hurriedly donned my clothes, anxiously hoping for a positive outcome. When I returned to the doctor's office, I found him standing by a large bookshelf adjacent to his desk, diligently searching through its contents. Several minutes elapsed before he located the specific book he sought. Leafing through its pages, he found what he searched for and paused to read it. I watched his expression become one of growing concern as he absorbed its contents. After a brief period, he returned to his seat at the desk, holding the book in his hands.

The weighty silence in the office was punctuated by the steady tick-tock of the clock hanging on the wall behind Dr. Sideman's chair. I scrutinized his face, searching for any hints that could offer insight into what he was about to reveal. His avoidance of eye contact only heightened my sense of apprehension, signaling that something was undeniably amiss. Gathering my courage, I mustered the strength to voice the question that weighed heavily on my heart, "Dr. Sideman, is there a problem with my baby?"

As I awaited Dr. Sideman's response, I gave myself a much-needed pep talk. I reminded myself this was the last prenatal visit of the year before Christmas. Focusing on the upcoming Christmas holiday filled me with childlike anticipation for the joyous moments awaiting my family. Christmas had always held a special place in my heart; now, as a mother, its significance had only deepened. I eagerly anticipate the holiday season—the joy of present shopping, the delight in decorating the Christmas tree, and our cherished tradition of opening one gift on Christmas Eve while savoring hot chocolate with marshmallows. Most of all, I eagerly await the sheer delight on my children's faces as they unwrap their gifts.

Amid such a beautiful time of year, what could possibly go wrong? With three successful pregnancies behind me, I had allowed a sense of confidence to settle in. I couldn't fathom anything derailing this journey.

DIAGNOSIS: CONGENITAL DIAPHRAGMATIC HERNIA

Amidst my racing thoughts, I was startled when Dr. Sideman called my name, "Mrs. Ebanks!" It snapped me out of my reverie, reminding me I was in his office, awaiting some serious news. Taking a deep breath, I steeled myself for what was to come.

With a grave tone, Dr. Sideman began, "There is a significant issue with your baby's development." Leaning forward, he used a pencil to trace an outline on the sonogram print resting on his desk. He explained that he had observed an anomaly during the second ultrasound scan. His pencil moved across the image as he spoke, highlighting various points. Although it appeared as scribbles and blotches, he identified specific areas as the baby's lungs, heart, and intestines. He then drew attention to another region, describing it as the presence of fluids. Dr. Sideman's voice carried a weight of concern as he said, "The root cause behind these occurrences is a birth defect caused by a congenital diaphragmatic hernia in your baby. This condition arises because of a hole in the diaphragm, the muscle that separates the chest cavity from the abdominal cavity. During fetal development, your baby's positioning in the womb has allowed the intestines to herniate or push through this hole, leading them to rest in the chest cavity. Consequently, this displacement has also shifted the heart toward the right side of your baby's body. Furthermore, this displacement has had an impact on the growth and maturation of his left lung. The space where the left lung should normally develop has become occupied by fluid, which is now hindering its proper formation."

Confusion and fear flooded my mind as I struggled to grasp what this all meant. *Was my baby going to die?* Recognizing my apprehension, Dr. Sideman finally locked eyes with me, his expression brimming with empathy. Speaking calmly and deliberately, he conveyed the gravity of the situation, emphasizing that, throughout his extensive career, this was the first time he had encountered this condition in his patients. As the weight of his words sank in, I didn't know how to respond.

He explained that the condition occurs during fetal development, and without proper management and intervention, my baby could experience respiratory challenges after birth.

The treatment for CDH takes place after the baby is born and typically involves a surgical procedure. During this surgery, surgeons work to restore the abdominal organs to their rightful place within the abdominal cavity and repair the hole in the diaphragm. In some cases, additional measures may be necessary, such as using extracorporeal membrane oxygenation (ECMO), a heart-lung bypass machine, to support the baby's breathing and circulation during and after the surgical intervention[4].

I was utterly overwhelmed by the information, my mind in turmoil. Panic surged through me, and I was so consumed by the gravity of what I'd just been told that I completely missed the doctor's mention of "his breathing." The revelation of the baby's gender didn't register until later that evening, as my sole and all-encompassing concern was his mortality.

Dr. Sideman sensed my anxiety and paused, leaning closer to convey his next steps. With a reassuring tone, he explained that we would need to register with the University Hospital of the West Indies (UHWI), the only hospital equipped with a neonatal intensive care unit (NICU) located below the delivery ward. This was crucial to ensure that my child would receive the immediate and specialized care necessary for his survival.

I arranged to collect the referral letter the first week in January. As I left the doctor's office, I became aware of Robert's presence. I was so deeply absorbed in shock that I hadn't even considered how this news might have impacted Robert. In somber silence, we made our way to the car. I felt a sense of relief that

---

4 "Congenital diaphragmatic hernia," CDH International, accessed February 2, 2023, **https://cdhi.org/what-is-congenital-diaphragmatic-hernia.**

we had chosen to share a vehicle that day, sparing me the added difficulty of returning to collect my own car after receiving such devastating news. My sole desire was to reach the comfort of my home, where I could begin the private process of coming to terms with the situation.

The news of the diagnosis weighed heavily on both of us. I could see Robert was worried, yet I felt powerless to offer comfort or reassurance. Trapped within the relentless grip of isolation and despair, I struggled to find a way to ease our burdens. I knew we needed support but wasn't sure where to turn.

LIGHT IN THE DARKNESS

In that moment of uncertainty, a familiar Bible verse echoed in my mind, "I praise you because I am fearfully and wonderfully made; your works are wonderful, I know that full well" (Psalm 139:14, NIV). Clinging to those words like a lifeline, I knew we needed support from our church's nurture leaders, Dave and Cathy, who lived nearby. I shared my thoughts with Robert, and he agreed.

Dave answered the phone on the first ring. He listened attentively as I explained our situation. Without hesitation, he invited Robert and me to visit their home that evening for a prayer session. Grateful for their support, we arrived at their doorstep at the agreed-upon time, and they welcomed us with open arms.

Cathy whisked me away in one direction while Dave took Robert aside. After some time, we reconvened in their cozy living room. Cathy shared a deeply personal story about one of their daughters, who had faced troubling test results as a toddler. She spoke candidly about their challenges and how their faith had been tested. She shared the strategies that had helped them cope, such as reading select Bible verses about healing over their daughter as she slept. Eventually, they found a medical facility in Canada that assisted them, and their daughter was now a college sophomore. Hearing their story, which mirrored our own in many ways, felt like a ray of light amidst the darkness. That day, we were greatly encouraged and reminded that we were not alone. They prayed for us, and we carried hope and strength as we left their home.

The Christmas festivities pushed the weight of the diagnosis into the background. But as January rolled in, the diagnosis resurfaced with new worries. *Would I be accepted at UHWI?* Their practice was to register mothers within the first six weeks of pregnancy. I was four months pregnant.

Securing a place in UHWI's maternity unit was a turning point. I had prayed for a miracle as I left home that day. However, I was worried when I arrived at the hospital and saw that I was the only visibly pregnant mother. The nurse on duty appeared surprised by my condition. After collecting my referral letter, she carefully observed me and my protruding belly before disappearing into the office behind the desk. After what felt like an eternity of anticipation, the nurse reappeared, holding a ticket in her hand. As she handed it to me, a wave of relief washed over me, knowing that I had been accepted as a private patient under the care of Dr. Sideman. It was a pivotal moment that brought a glimmer of hope amidst the uncertainties we faced.

In the days that followed, I discovered that our baby's CDH diagnosis had played an unexpected role in our acceptance. The clinicians found our case intriguing and were eager to study and treat it. It was as if the very condition that had caused us so much worry had now become an advantage, working in our favor. I couldn't help but see it as a divine intervention, a testament to God's grace and providence in our lives.

TAKEAWAY

This experience touched me deeply on multiple levels. It reminded me of life's unpredictable nature and its lack of guarantees. It demonstrated firsthand how circumstances can swiftly shift, leaving us in a state of fear and uncertainty.

But, amid all the uncertainty, it became abundantly clear that we were not alone. Unbeknownst to us initially, Dave and Cathy had traveled a similar path, and as mature believers and parents, they were right there when we needed them to encourage and support us. The likelihood of us being acquainted with them, living close to them, and being members of the nurture group they led seemed almost serendipitous. This was a sign of the divine intervention that was guiding us along our path. That day ended up being a powerful source of encouragement, fortifying my faith.

CHAPTER 4

THE BIRTH OF THIS GIFT FROM GOD

A Series of False Starts

Despite receiving the diagnosis, I clung to the hope that everything would turn out well when my baby was born. I held firmly to the belief that this child was a gift from God; therefore, I anticipated a seamless journey. Having now registered with UHWI, I thought the worst was over. Looking back, I realize I had crafted a narrative around this belief—a narrative of miracles, divine healing, and an uncomplicated delivery. I had never entertained the thought that things could take a different course.

I had my first prenatal appointment at UHWI a week later, and Robert accompanied me. As we were wrapping up the appointment, a nurse asked if we were familiar with the location of the delivery unit. Given that it was my first appointment, we hadn't yet had a chance to explore. She kindly suggested we tour the unit before departing and even provided directions.

Taking her advice, we set out to find the unit. Having Robert with me on this visit was comforting, and I started believing that things had leveled off. Little did I know that the challenges we had faced so far were merely a prelude to what lay ahead. The calm I felt in that moment was fleeting, for an even greater storm was about to descend upon us.

Later that night, I was abruptly awakened by intense abdominal pain, a clear indication that I was experiencing premature labor. The sensation was all too familiar to me. I had previously endured premature labor with Ryan and Jordanne. Ryan arrived after two false starts at thirty-three and a half weeks, while Jordanne had three false alarms before finally making her debut at thirty-five weeks.

Despite providing this crucial information to my ob-gyn, it somehow failed to make its way into my health records. This experience was significant as it marked the earliest point in any of my pregnancies when I had gone into labor, as I was just five months pregnant. I was particularly concerned because Dr. Sideman had emphasized the importance of carrying the baby as close to full term as possible. Doing so would significantly improve the chances of a successful congenital diaphragmatic hernia (CDH) repair surgery after he was born.

We promptly arranged for a neighbor to stay with the children until their grandparents arrived to pick them up, and then hurried to the hospital. Upon our arrival, I was swiftly processed and attended to. The medical team administered medication to arrest the advancement of labor, aiming to prolong the pregnancy and secure the best possible outcome for both the baby and me. I remained under observation for several days to ensure the cessation of labor, and it was only when the medical team confirmed my stability that I was discharged and allowed to return home. However, ongoing caution and the need for follow-up care remained essential.

Shortly after returning to work, I dove headfirst into organizing a major corporate event, which I eventually executed in Montego Bay a month later. It soon became apparent that I had overexerted myself with the project when I was awakened once again in the early morning, wracked with labor pains.

At the hospital, I met with Dr. Sideman, who promptly initiated a series of tests, among them an ultrasound, to evaluate the situation. The ultrasound findings were concerning, as they unveiled a cervical tear and indicated two centimeters of dilation, clearly presenting a significant risk to the baby's ability to remain securely in place.

Despite the significant risks associated with my advanced stage of pregnancy, Dr. Sideman presented a daring proposal: a cerclage[5] procedure to stitch my cervix. As we deliberated, the weight of the decision hung heavy in the room. We understood that this surgery offered our greatest hope of extending the pregnancy, and with determined hearts, we gave our consent.

I remained under close monitoring for ten days during that hospital stay to ensure my stability. To promote my baby's lung development, I received two rounds of steroid shots, specifically corticosteroids. As my doctor explained, these shots consist of synthetic hormones designed to expedite the development of the baby's lungs and other crucial organs.

The two doses of the shots, administered twenty-four hours apart, proved to be remarkably painful. The discomfort lingered

---

5 A cerclage is a surgical procedure performed on a pregnant mother to help prevent premature birth or pregnancy loss. It involves stitching or suturing the cervix closed to support and stabilize the uterus during pregnancy.

long after my son's birth, and it took several months for the injection site to finally ease its persistent soreness. On the tenth day, I was discharged and sent home on a full bed rest order.

However, that wasn't the end of my challenges. I experienced premature labor twice by the time I reached the eight-month mark in my pregnancy. During the latter of these hospitalizations, my doctor happened to be away attending a medical conference. Exhausted and drained, I drifted to sleep as the contractions slowly subsided.

While I was in the hospital, going through the necessary monitoring to prevent my pregnancy from ending prematurely and to ensure my baby stayed in position, an unexpected and rather bizarre incident occurred.

Out of the blue, a young resident doctor barged into my room without so much as a greeting or a question. He immediately began examining me, his actions startling and abrupt. Before I could even process what was happening, he reached for a pair of scissors and unceremoniously cut the sutures that were supposed to hold for several more weeks. I was utterly bewildered and anxious, and I asked him why he had done such a thing since I wasn't yet due. I was only eight months pregnant.

Taken aback, he glanced at the chart he had brought with him into the room. He hesitantly asked if I wasn't Ms. Green. With a calm but firm tone, I corrected him and gave him my actual name. He looked embarrassed and uttered an awkward "oops" before hastily retreating from the room. Interestingly, who it was remained a mystery since he didn't put this information in my patient file, and I didn't get his name.

This unsettling encounter served as a profound wake-up call, highlighting the importance of vigilance in navigating the health-care system. Until then, I had been fortunate to have only good healthcare and delivery experiences. So, the concept of medical self-advocacy hadn't registered with me.

AWAKENING TO PATIENT ADVOCACY

However, this experience forcefully opened my eyes to the imperative need for active participation in my healthcare jour-ney. It was a revelation that illuminated the significance of em-powerment for all patients, enabling them to communicate with providers and be actively involved in decision-making concern-ing their own health and that of their loved ones.

Moreover, I realized that if I had been more vigilant, asking questions when the resident entered my room, it could have had the potential to prevent errors, ensure personalized care, and pri-oritize my and my baby's safety.

Upon being discharged, I became acutely aware of my vul-nerability at this crucial stage of my pregnancy. Without the re-assurance of the cerclage, I had to take every possible measure to remain still and reduce potential risks. As a result, I completely stopped working and dedicated my time to rest in bed. This pe-riod also gave me much-needed time for conversations, Bible reading, and journaling.

In addition, I had the joy of being "held captive" by my chil-dren, who were delighted that I was always at home. They knew exactly where to find me and seized the opportunity to entertain me with their jokes, lively accounts of their school day, off-key songs, and stories composed just for the baby. They were delight-ed to join me in bed, play quietly, or share the space with their beloved toys. It proved to be an enjoyable and memorable way to spend my bed rest, and almost before I knew it, the thirty-seventh week arrived, accompanied by my doctor's consent to resume mobility gradually. This milestone marked the baby's sufficient development to enter the world safely.

THE BIRTH

At the stroke of midnight in the thirty-seventh week of my pregnancy, I awoke to find myself drenched in bed. My water had broken, signaling the imminent arrival of my long-awaited baby. With a sense of urgency, we swiftly made our way to the hospital, having become seasoned experts in navigating this process. However, the re-emergence of concerns related to the congenital diaphragmatic hernia diagnosis brought a renewed wave of anxiety and apprehension, intensifying the already tense atmosphere.

I was lying in the labor ward bed when that first wave of pain hit me. It was so sudden and intense that it felt as though all the pain from my three previous pregnancies had returned at once, merging with the current agony of delivery.

At that moment, I was acutely aware of the toll that the multiple false starts had taken on me, both physically and mentally, and emotionally. I felt utterly drained, and the prospect of facing the challenges of this delivery seemed daunting and overwhelming. Alongside these intense sensations, there crept in a growing awareness and fear that I might not have the strength to go through with a natural birth.

However, I soon realized I had little control over the situation as the delivery unfolded with remarkable speed. In my overwhelming desperation, I turned to prayer, seeking strength and divine help, as I feared I might not make it through.

To my surprise and comfort, I felt a gentle touch on my shoulder, almost as if it were an answer to my prayer. As I opened my eyes, I was met with the comforting presence of a compassionate older nurse. Her warm countenance and soothing touch immediately calmed my racing heart.

She shared with me that her shift was coming to a close, but upon seeing me, she felt an irresistible urge to approach. With a sincere and caring tone, she asked how I was doing, and I didn't hold back—I let her know that I was truly struggling. In an immensely compassionate gesture, she asked if I would like her to stay with me for a while. I was grateful for her companionship, so I quickly agreed. I was still alone at that moment; Robert had left to find a parking spot after dropping me off and hadn't returned yet.

Gently, she rested her hand on my belly. As another contraction rolled in, she encouraged me to breathe deeply, but I confessed that I was unfamiliar with the techniques. Despite having gone through three pregnancies and deliveries before, I had never attended a Lamaze class, so I had no idea how to follow her advice.

Sensing my difficulty, the nurse took an unorthodox but deeply empathetic approach. She softly laid her hand on my belly and began to pray. It was a gesture that revealed an intuitive understanding of what I needed at that moment. It was as though she instinctively knew that prayer would bring me a sense of calm and reassurance.

While I couldn't hear the exact words, I watched her lips move earnestly as she reached out to a higher power. The effect of her prayer was profound, enveloping both me and my baby in a soothing sense of tranquility.

Before her prayer, it felt as if my little one was restless, almost like he was trying to break free. However, his movements became more purposeful and aligned with the birthing process as he responded to the faith-activated support surrounding us. It was a profound transformation, and I felt deep gratitude for the nurse's understanding, compassion, and ability to provide the spiritual comfort I needed to endure.

Guided by her calming presence, the nurse led me through breathing exercises, teaching me techniques to alleviate the intensity of the pain. Robert had arrived, and with him holding my hand and each guided breath, I tapped into a newfound reserve of strength to navigate the challenges of labor. I fell asleep after a while.

I was abruptly jolted awake by an intense surge of pain, indicating that I had entered the final stages of labor. Beside me, Robert sat quietly, his concerned presence offering a small measure of comfort. However, the kind nurse who provided support earlier left for the night, leaving me feeling vulnerable and trepidatious. As the pains continued with increasing force, a wave of desperation and fear washed over me, signaling that something was amiss.

I called out desperately for a nurse to assist me, but none came. Sensing my distress, Robert left in search of help, leaving me alone to face this critical moment. I could feel the baby's movement, but amidst my echoing cries for help reverberating through the room, the silence persisted; no one came.

Finally, I summoned every ounce of remaining strength and

called again, "Nurse! The baby is coming!" At that instance, a short, elderly woman burst through the curtains, muttering that I was making noise for no good reason. She said I had been checked an hour before and was not ready to deliver. But I implored her to check again, as I could feel the baby descending. I told her I had precipitous labor[6] with all three of my previous pregnancies. Even though I had informed my doctor about my history of rapid labor and the associated concerns, regrettably, this crucial information was not included in my birth plan. There were no preparations in place to address this development—it caught everyone off guard. To add to the complexity, my doctor was not present when it happened, which left the nurse attending to me feeling understandably overwhelmed and slightly panicked.

This new information immediately grabbed her attention, prompting her to act swiftly. She began to check me, all the while muttering that I wasn't yet ready to deliver. But as she checked me, I could feel her body tensing with a newfound sense of urgency. Reacting promptly, she called for a porter to transfer me to the delivery room. It was evident that I had entered the final stage of labor. The room erupted into a flurry of activities as preparations were made for my transfer, and all the while, Robert stood on the side, looking on helplessly.

I was transferred to the delivery room and settled onto the bed, but once again, the nurse left me alone. Minutes passed, and I could sense the baby descending into the birthing canal. I called out for a nurse in my urgency, but there was no response. As the baby's head emerged, a surge of panic gripped me, and I cried out for the nurse once more. Unbeknownst to me, Robert anxiously waited outside the room, later recounting the nurse's

6 Precipitous labor is characterized by an unusually fast progression of labor, from the onset of contractions to the birth of the baby, typically lasting less than three hours.

frantic efforts to find any available doctor, as none were present on the floor.

I was in the midst of a painful and urgent moment, but the nurse remained in denial, repeatedly murmuring that I wasn't ready to deliver. That's when Robert stepped in, his worry for our well-being overriding his patience. He firmly told her he wouldn't hesitate to take legal action against the hospital if anything went wrong with me or the baby. This ultimatum finally got her to reenter the room and take the situation seriously.

She reentered the room just as Nathan started making his way into the world. Upon seeing that he was already crowning, she urgently told me to close my legs in an attempt to delay the birth, explaining that a doctor was still on the way. But despite her frantic efforts, my son arrived just a few minutes later, precisely at 4:25 a.m. on May 4, 2004.

Regrettably, none of the provisions in my birthing plan were carried out. The plan specifically stated that due to the baby's diaphragmatic hernia and his underdeveloped left lung, he should be placed in an incubator before the umbilical cord was cut. In the chaos of the delivery, this crucial step was either overlooked or omitted.

A Chaotic Arrival: Navigating the Unexpected in the Delivery Room

A sudden flurry of activity erupted in the delivery room as the neonatal intensive care unit (NICU) team rushed in. With swift precision, they began the vital task of stabilizing the baby. Unfortunately, there was no incubator available in the room as per my birth plan. However, they skillfully improvised by manually administering the necessary oxygen as they prepared to transfer him to the NICU located downstairs.

Amidst the overwhelming chaos, I felt forgotten as I strained to catch a glimpse of my baby or hear his cry. But there was only silence. The team worked diligently, seemingly oblivious to my presence, which was quite distressing. Just as swiftly as they had arrived, they left with my baby.

The matron quietly reappeared and attended to my immediate post-delivery needs with a sense of detached efficiency. She did not make eye contact as she prepared me for the next steps. She briefly mentioned that my doctor would visit later and promptly called for a porter to transfer me to the post-delivery unit.

I lay in a daze, struggling to make sense of what had just happened. This birth experience was far from what I had envisioned, especially given the extensive preparation we had undertaken beforehand. In that critical delivery moment, it felt as though everything had fallen apart. I couldn't help but wonder, *What did all of this mean?*

TAKEAWAY

I went into labor with the strong conviction that I was welcoming a child blessed as a "gift" by God. I believed this would mean a straightforward journey, but reality proved otherwise. This was my first experience giving birth in a public hospital, leaving me uncertain if the ensuing chaos was a personal anomaly. What I am certain of, however, is that it left a deep emotional scar that haunted me for years. It took me a long time to revisit that experience without tearing up or feeling angry.

But, as the years have passed, I came out on the other end of the experience, understanding that uncovering meaning and purpose amid adversity is a deeply personal and individual process that requires time, reflection, and a deep connection to faith and spirituality. Through these lenses, I now see the blessings: from the off-duty nurse who sat with me and helped me in my darkest hour to Robert standing up for our baby and me when I couldn't to the safe delivery of my child. Indeed, it was nothing short of a miracle that we emerged from this experience stronger and more appreciative, knowing that God was with us through it all.

CHAPTER 5

POST-DELIVERY REALITIES

Life after a CDH Birth

It was a while before I found myself in the post-delivery unit, a mixture of anxiety and bewilderment swirling within me. No one had provided any explanations, not even regarding my baby's condition. My doctor had yet to appear, and the uncertainty about my child left me deeply worried. As the day progressed, I remained unattended in the unit, feeling as though I had been forgotten.

As I surveyed my temporary surroundings, I couldn't help but notice that the space resembled a large auditorium. It was lined with rows upon rows of beds instead of seats, each enclosed by a flimsy curtain offering only a fragile illusion of privacy within this shared space. For most of the day, the curtains were drawn back, exposing each patient to the gaze of everyone in and who entered the ward. I felt exposed and vulnerable in that open environment. No one seemed to care.

As I settled into my designated bed, my eyes roamed the room, noting that each bed was occupied, and mothers either held their newborns or had the baby beside them in the bassinet.

The enormity of it all washed over me, and I could not stem the tears. Amidst the bustling atmosphere of the unit, I sat alone, consumed by an overwhelming sense of defeat. No one, not even the nurses, spared a moment to check in on me, leaving me to deal with my anguish alone.

I drifted off to sleep and was roused by Robert's arrival. He was in the NICU and assured me that our baby was alive. He said my doctor had finally arrived and would visit me soon. We sat in silence, awaiting his arrival.

In the midafternoon, my doctor finally showed up, but the rapport we had established during the months of prenatal visits had dissipated. He seemed evasive, and a sense of unease filled the air, replacing the trust I once had in him. The way events had unfolded left both of us unsettled. Swiftly, he conducted his examinations, granting me clearance to be discharged the following day. Meanwhile, Robert needed to leave to pick up our other children from school, so we arranged to visit the NICU the next morning.

That night, I couldn't sleep well and eagerly awaited the morning. With nothing else to occupy my attention, I became fixated on the tender moments between the nearby mothers and their babies. I noticed something peculiar during one of my trips to the bathroom at the end of the hallway. The mothers closest to me seemed to be watching me closely. To my surprise, they reacted swiftly, hastily gathering their babies and giving me suspicious glances. Confused by their behavior, I approached one of the nurses for an explanation.

That's when I learned about a disheartening reality that often exists in local public hospitals. Some mothers who had experienced the devastating loss of their own babies would occasionally attempt to steal another newborn. It was a shocking revelation, and I felt appalled and disheartened to realize that without knowing anything about my circumstances or myself, I was being perceived as a potential threat—a baby-stealer, no less.

Following that encounter, I made a conscious effort to avert my gaze and avoided making eye contact with any of the other mothers. This only deepened my sense of isolation in the bustling environment around me.

MEETING MY BABY FOR THE FIRST TIME

The following morning finally arrived, and together with Robert, we made our way to the NICU to visit our newborn son. As we arrived at the unit, the nurse stationed near the entrance discreetly directed us toward a small door at the room's rear. The NICU was relatively spacious, with rows of small bassinets, each cradling a delicate infant. We made our way to the back of the room and entered through the designated door. Inside, there were four large, sterile incubation units, and three of them were occupied by infants.

I approached the trio of incubators with a sense of trepidation, realizing that I had never met my own baby and was unsure which one belonged to us. Just as panic threatened to take hold, Robert reached out and gently touched my hand, directing my attention to one of the units which was labeled "Baby Ebanks."

As I laid my eyes on my son, a wave of emotions overwhelmed me. My knees gave way, and I instinctively clung to Robert. What I saw took me completely by surprise. His tiny body, weighing only five pounds and five ounces, was entangled within a complex network of tubes enclosed within an intimidating and oversized machine. Intravenous lines snaked their way into his delicate hands and legs while nasal gastric tubes were inserted in both nostrils. A catheter was visibly protruding from his diaper, and to add to the overwhelming sight, a tube extended from his left chest, suctioning fluids from his lungs. The upper half of his face was covered with a bandage, securing the nasal gastric tubes in place. My heart couldn't help but ache for my son as I imagined the discomfort and perhaps pain he was going through.

That was the moment when the full weight of my son's condition crashed down upon me, a tidal wave of dizziness and helplessness sweeping over me. I felt utterly powerless, disoriented by the stark reality before us—our child was born with CHD. Robert and I held onto each other tightly, our hands interlocked, as we confronted the daunting truth of our son's situation.

I was dismayed at the realization of the difficulty he now faced. I wasn't sure he would make it. I couldn't fathom how a child of promise, a gift of God, could have this terrible experience. From the moment he nestled in my womb, it appeared he had been engaged in a relentless battle for the simple right to exist. And now, as we faced the harsh reality, he was handed a precarious fifty-fifty chance at survival. As I contemplated the uncertain road ahead, I didn't know if I could survive.

The surgeon joined us and finally offered the first substantial information about our son since birth. She carefully explained that they had effectively stabilized our son the previous night.

Their intention was to monitor his condition closely for another day, and if all continued to improve as expected, the surgery would be scheduled for the day after.

Shortly after the visit, I was discharged from the hospital. The drive home felt eerily quiet, a reflection of the heavy emotions weighing on my heart. It was as though I had just completed a grueling marathon, only to find myself without the victor's trophy. The weight of disappointment and disillusionment pressed down on my soul, casting a deep shadow of desolation that enveloped me entirely. I felt as if I were sinking, consumed by it all.

Adding to my despair was the sight of my older children waiting eagerly for my return, their eyes filled with expectation. I felt guilty that we had forgotten to explain the true nature of their brother's illness and why he wouldn't be coming home with me. I tried to explain it as best as possible, but I could see them fighting back the tears.

That evening, I couldn't bear to meet Robert's gaze, for I carried the weight of failure for our son and him. Sleep remained elusive as I settled into bed that night; my mind, a whirlwind of restless thoughts. In the quiet hours before dawn, tormented by my inner turmoil, I turned to prayer. I pleaded with God, a desperate reminder of His promise concerning our child. The stakes were high, not just for our son's well-being but also for the very bedrock of my faith in God.

TAKEAWAY

The entire sequence of events—from my son's birth to how communication was handled within the hospital and among the medical team—left me deeply traumatized. I found myself grap-

RAISING NATHAN, AGAINST ALL ODDS

pling with the inexplicable question of why this was unfolding within my family. Despite being aware of my baby's condition, I remained unprepared for the stark and painful reality it brought about.

It took time for me to process the complex emotions I had carried, including acknowledging this trauma. It was years before I could talk about these experiences without falling apart. But talking and writing about it were pivotal in my journey toward healing. Giving myself the permission to express my true emotions opened the door to understanding, acceptance, and personal growth.

CHAPTER 6

CHALLENGING FATE: CONFRONTING THE ODDS

Countdown to Surgery

The next morning, a heavy and somber atmosphere filled the air as I prepared my older children for school. Little did I realize at the time that their brother's hospitalization was impacting them too. They were still very young, and I was unaware of this aspect. Even if I had recognized it, I wouldn't have known how to address their emotions because I was traveling in uncharted territory.

Despite the mood, we tried to maintain a sense of normalcy in our daily routine. Robert took the children to school before going to work, while I, officially on maternity leave from work, went to the hospital. I was anxious as I didn't know if my baby survived the night.

The commute to the hospital felt especially lengthy due to heavy traffic, which only aggravated my discomfort. Upon finally securing a parking spot in the hospital's lot, I was confronted with another source of worry—the daunting trek from the parking lot to the neonatal intensive care unit (NICU). As I stepped out of the minivan, a sharp twinge of pain made me wince involuntarily. Every muscle in my body seemed to ache with each movement, amplifying my exhaustion, weariness, muscle soreness, and general physical discomfort. The long drive had only intensified the fatigue I was already grappling with, having given birth just a few days before.

To make matters worse, the extended period of sitting had aggravated my postpartum pains and discomfort, adding to my overall physical unease. Despite these challenges, the thought of seeing my baby kept me going.

Upon entering the unit, a wave of relief washed over me, but my physical state painted a different picture. I gasped for breath, my body drenched in a cold sweat, and my heart raced within my chest. An unrelenting headache had plagued me since delivering my son, and my blood pressure was elevated.

It took me a while to catch my breath, only to have it snatched away again when I saw my baby. In the harsh light of day, he looked very sick, almost as if he was hanging on to life by a thread. At two days old, his eyes were still closed, and he seemed oblivious to the world around him. Surrounding his incubator were three other units, with newborns on either side of him, each engaged in their own courageous struggle for survival.

Despite my best efforts, tears streamed down my cheeks uncontrollably as I sat beside his incubator, overwhelmed by the gripping fear of losing him. The steady hum and beeps emanating from the machines only intensified my anxiety, as I was unfamiliar with their meaning.

Whenever the monitors sounded an alarm, a tight grip of panic seized me, causing my heart to race in response to the jarring sounds. Sometimes, a nurse would calmly enter the room, swiftly resolving the issue and silencing the beeping, providing momentary relief. Other times, a small team would rush in and usher me out. The uncertainty of the situation heightened the gravity of each beep, causing it to feel like a looming threat. I would instinctively brace myself for the worst, my anxiety intensifying with every sound.

It took me a while to discern whether my baby's monitor had gone off amidst the cacophony. However, even when I did, it did little to alleviate my anxiety, as it felt as if the struggles and challenges of the other parents and their babies resonated deep within me. Their fears and hopes mirrored my own, creating an unspoken bond between us all.

Later that morning, the surgeon arrived to discuss the upcoming CDH surgery. I felt a mix of relief that the procedure could finally take place and fear about what it entailed. It was difficult to receive this news independently, without any support. Nonetheless, I focused on listening attentively, determined to grasp all shared information.

The surgeon explained that since my baby had been stable for over forty-eight hours, they had scheduled the surgery for the following day. She detailed the procedure, starting with the administration of general anesthesia to ensure my baby's comfort and unconsciousness throughout the surgery. Then, the surgical team would make an incision, typically on the side of the chest or abdomen, to gain access to the diaphragm. Carefully, they would relocate the abdominal organs that had herniated into his chest back into their proper place within the abdominal cavity.

The subsequent phase entailed the repair of the diaphragmatic hole. The surgeon outlined different techniques that could be employed, including suturing the edges of the diaphragm or utilizing a patch to reinforce the repair. She emphasized that the choice of treatment depended on the size and location of the defect, so a final decision couldn't be made until they were inside him. Nevertheless, once the repair was executed, the medical team would meticulously examine the integrity of the diaphragm and ensure the correct positioning of the organs before concluding the procedure by closing the incision with stitches.

As the surgeon spoke with a detached, matter-of-fact tone, each word landed on me like a sharp blow. I struggled to absorb the vast amount of information, worry, and fear that filled the room. When she finally finished, she asked me if I had any questions. However, I was so overwhelmed by the weight of it all that I couldn't think clearly.

Amidst the whirlwind of thoughts, one question managed to break through the chaos: *Would he survive?* But I was paralyzed by fear, unable to voice such a haunting possibility. *What if uttering those words aloud makes them real?* I couldn't take that chance, so I said I had no questions.

Following our conversation, she handed me the consent papers, briefly explaining their purpose. As I mechanically went through the motions of signing those documents, each pen stroke carried the weight of immense responsibility. With every stroke of the pen, it felt like I was relinquishing a fragment of my hope for my baby's survival. The weight of the decision pressed heavily upon me as I grappled with the reality of entrusting my child's life to the care of others. It was a poignant reminder of my vulnerability as a parent and the immense trust I had to place in the medical team to do what was best for my little one.

NAVIGATING THE TURBULENT WATERS OF THE NICU

As the surgeon walked away, I remained behind, alone with my jumbled emotions and contemplative thoughts. The beeping sounds of the machines kept me company as they punctuated the quiet of the room. I felt adrift, desperately yearning for someone to lean on, someone who could share the burden and provide comfort and encouragement. I wanted to reach out to Robert; however, the strict no cell phone policy in the NICU would mean walking outside to the parking lot. I didn't have the strength to do so and was in intense physical pain. So, instead, I sat in silence. In that quiet space, I prayed.

In the early evening, I was joined by the other babies' mothers in the room. We each sat next to our baby, enveloped in our own worries. Just as I stood up to leave for the day, a sudden and sharp piercing beep shattered the air emanating from one of the incubators. In an instant, events unfolded rapidly, making it impossible to discern which baby was in crisis. Amidst the flurry of activity, several nurses rushed into the room, and we were quickly ushered out. Doctors rushed in, and medical personnel went in and out of the room for a brief while. All the while, I stood a short distance from the door in a huddle with the other two mothers as we tried to figure out what was happening.

After what felt like a long wait, a nurse emerged and beckoned to one of the parents standing next to me. I was overcome with relief that it wasn't my baby. But as I heard the loud wail of the mother coming from the room, I realized the child had passed away. I cried along with her, as did some of the other mothers in the outside unit. As we grieved with her, I realized that, but for God's grace, that could have been my child.

I reluctantly left the hospital to go home that night. As soon as I exited the building, I called Robert and shared what had happened, including the planned procedure for the next morning. I could sense that he, too, was deeply emotional about everything. He left work early that day and canceled his class to sit with our son.

By the time I arrived home, I felt physically unwell. It became evident that the weight of the situation and the physical demands of the day had exacted their toll on me. This was amplified by the fact that I had spent the entire day by my son's side without consuming any food or water.

However, my children—Adrianne, Ryan, and Jordanne—were still awake, anxiously awaiting news about their little brother. The guilt I felt was overwhelming as I told them he wouldn't be coming home. Explaining the impending surgery posed another challenge I wasn't prepared for. I could see how they were trying to muster their courage, which was heart-wrenching.

As they finally settled into bed for the night, I found myself mentally and emotionally drained, with physical exhaustion compounding my state. I sat alone in the dark of my bedroom and cried. It was too much, and I didn't know how I would manage the surgery the next day. *What if he didn't make it?* It was hard to be hopeful when everything felt like it was going wrong. But giving up was not an option for me, so I kept praying. That night was the beginning of an ongoing struggle with acute insomnia that would last for several months.

TAKEAWAY

The primary lesson I learned through the experiences described in this chapter is how profoundly influential a child's medical crisis can be on an entire family, including young siblings. Nothing or no one prepared us for this, and this left us in the dark about how to support our children in such a situation. Furthermore, it became evident that the healthcare system itself appeared oblivious to the physical, mental, and emotional toll Robert and I, as parents, were enduring. Throughout this trying ordeal, we found no support or assistance to help us cope with our immense burden.

The second key point underscores the critical role of medical and healthcare professionals in assisting parents as they navigate this harrowing situation. In our experience, we encountered doctors who alternated between two extremes: providing us with an overwhelming flood of information that left us feeling bewildered or frustratingly withholding necessary information. Either of these could have pushed us to our breaking point. The shortcomings within the medical system compelled me to turn to my faith for the help and support I needed.

CHAPTER 7

THE CDH SURGERY

Preparation and Planning

My Christian upbringing and how I practiced my faith didn't fully prepare me for the daunting reality of my child undergoing a major surgery with potentially life-threatening implications. In the midst of my emotional turmoil, the thought of turning to my faith community didn't even cross my mind. However, I instinctively turned to my daily practice of reading the Bible and praying to start my day.

On that day, my personal connection with God, as nurtured by the words of Psalm 118:17 (NIV), "I will not die but live, and will proclaim what the Lord has done," became my steadfast anchor. I poured out my deepest concerns, fears, and hopes to God, expressing sincere gratitude for His deliverance of my child through the surgical ordeal and the incredible opportunity to bear witness to His miraculous works. In those moments of intense uncertainty, I found comfort and inner strength through deep contemplation of the verse, which revealed God's multifaceted nature—as the giver of life, the author of miracles, and the consistently reliable source of faithfulness and trustworthiness in my life.

I made a point to arrive at the hospital early to pray with my son before his surgery. The circumstances proved challenging, as only one parent was allowed in the NICU at a time, and I knew deep down that I needed Robert with me. Nevertheless, we had agreed that I would be the one to be there with him.

Shortly after I took my place beside my baby, the surgical team arrived and began their preparations. Aside from a brief morning greeting, they proceeded with their tasks as if I were invisible. No explanations were offered, and no information was shared. Uncertain of my role in that moment, I chose to remain silent, positioning myself in a corner where I could closely observe their every action without impeding their progress. As they meticulously organized everything, silent tears welled in my eyes as I prayed earnestly for the surgical team's skills and the procedure's success. I also tried to believe in my baby's ability to sense my presence and find comfort in the knowledge that he was not alone, even with his eyes closed.

As the moment approached for them to transfer my son to the operating theatre, my anxiety surged to new heights. They gently lifted him from the neonatal incubator,[7] and a nurse promptly secured an oxygen mask, enabling her to administer the required oxygen using a handheld pump. Concerns swirled through my mind as I envisioned the potential complications that could arise from the NICU to the operating theatre.

---

7 A medical device designed to create and maintain a controlled and sterile environment for newborn infants, especially premature or ill babies. This specialized apparatus provides a safe and temperature-controlled space to support the growth and health of neonates in a hospital setting.

Silently, they started pushing the gurney, taking my son away, and I stood there, torn. My heart ached to stay as close as possible to him, so I quietly followed them to the entrance of the operating theatre and stayed outside in adherence to their protocols. A short while later, security personnel approached me and informed me that no one was permitted to remain in that area. With a heavy heart and profound reluctance, I acquiesced to their instructions and slowly proceeded toward the waiting room on the upper floor.

With every step I took, the weight of anticipation, uncertainty, and an overwhelming sense of helplessness pressed upon me. The journey from the operating theatre's entrance to the waiting room seemed interminable, as if time itself had deliberately stretched to amplify the intensity of my emotions. The waiting room mirrored my inner turmoil, with subdued conversations and noticeable anxiety creating an environment that mirrored my own state of mind.

THE WAIT

As the life-threatening surgery for my baby's congenital diaphragmatic hernia (CDH) repair began, a fragile but steadfast hope hung in the air like a delicate thread. The surgical team's skilled hands tirelessly repaired the small breach in his diaphragm while the hospital's hallways buzzed with anxious energy. Inside the waiting room, a mix of emotions swirled within me—fear, faith, uncertainty, and gratitude. Each second on the clock seemed to echo through the room, intensifying the heavy silence and serving as a constant reminder of time passing. My heart, suspended in uncertainty, wrestled with the unfamiliar territory of maintaining hope amidst the unknown.

Every fiber of my being ached for the reassuring news that his surgery was proceeding smoothly. The mounting fear within me felt suffocating as if it were determined to steal my very breath. In that tense moment, my world seemed to hang in the balance, teetering on the edge of hope and despair. Each passing second intensified the emotional turmoil, making the need for positive updates all the more urgent.

My phone buzzed incessantly, overwhelmed with text messages from caring loved ones. Within the deluge of texts, a particular message stood out. It read, "He will not die but live to proclaim the glory of God." It was personalized from Psalm 118[8], but it would be some time before I would become aware that it was a scripture from the Bible. Nonetheless, I found consolation in those words. I noticed that this message came from an unknown phone number multiple times as if it was meant to reach me each time worry threatened to consume me. During the long wait, I would repeat those words to reassure myself: "He will not die but live." It became my mantra, a source of comfort that sustained me throughout the agonizing wait.

Finally, four hours after he was taken into surgery, the door to the unit swung open, and my heart leaped with relief as the head doctor for the NICU entered. Though she wasn't part of the surgical team, I greeted her eagerly, hoping she had some news. She did not but offered to check with surgery. As I waited for her return, I kept repeating the Bible verse, "Now faith is confidence in what we hope for and assurance about what we do not see."[9] It solidified the idea of entrusting our faith in God and relying on His promises, particularly in that critical moment when there was no tangible evidence to assure me that my son's surgery would

8 Psalm 118:17 (NIV)
9 Hebrews 11:1 (NIV)

be successful.

The doctor reappeared a short while later, explaining that the surgery had a delayed start but was proceeding well. It strengthened my resolve to stay hopeful.

Around an hour later, the lead surgeon summoned me, indicating that the surgery had come to an end. I rushed to her, nearly running, my heart pounding with anticipation, craving the news she had to share.

A Closer Look at the Procedure

The surgeon's expression was solemn as I entered the room. She invited me to take a seat and immediately launched into an explanation of the procedure. Her opening remark was, "The surgery went as well as could be expected." Although I wasn't entirely sure what that meant, I signaled for her to continue.

She went on to describe that the procedure was rather straightforward. They had performed the surgery by making an incision, gently relocating his intestines back into his stomach, and skillfully sealing the hole in his diaphragm with minimal blood loss.

I began expressing my gratitude, but she raised her hand to indicate she had more to share. She continued by explaining that due to the size of the hole in his diaphragm, they needed to introduce a new material to seal it. Her next words sent shockwaves through my body, "This carries the risk of compatibility issues, as his body might recognize the material as foreign and potentially reject it. Additionally, because we had to handle his intestines when we pushed them back into place, there's a chance that his body may also reject the areas we touched, and they may wither and die. So, that is why I said we have to wait and see how he responds before we can know if the surgery was successful."

She maintained a clinical and matter-of-fact demeanor as she spoke, seemingly unaware of her words' profound impact on me. I instinctively shut out her words as I fought to keep my composure and avoid succumbing to despair. I couldn't bear to listen any further, fearing it might push me over the emotional precipice. That was the moment I gave her a fitting nickname—Dr. Doom.

Upon his return to the incubator, I was confronted with more trauma. A sizable bandage now adorned the middle of his fragile body, its width running from his chest to his lower abdomen. He now had even more tubes and wires than before. Among them was a large total parenteral nutrition (TPN) line, which I learned was a method of delivering complete nutrition intravenously to individuals unable to obtain adequate nourishment through oral feeding. This way, a balanced mixture of nutrients would be sent directly into the bloodstream, bypassing his stomach[10].

The realization struck me that my son had not been fed since birth due to his inability to process food or drink because of CDH. He had been hungry for three days. Since his body needed to heal, the doctor couldn't provide a definite timeframe for when he would be fed.

I didn't know how much more I could take. The relentless barrage of challenges had left me feeling emotionally drained and on the verge of breaking. As I sat looking at my son, a conversation with Cathy resurfaced in my mind. Back when we had first received the devastating CDH diagnosis, Cathy and her husband Dave had confided in Robert and me about how they had

---

10   KK Maudar, "Total Parenteral Nutrition," Medical Journal Armed Forces India 51, no. 2 (1995): 122-126, **https://doi.org/10.1016/S0377-1237(17)30942-5**.

found strength in Bible verses on healing when their daughter faced her own medical struggles.

So, right there in the NICU, I looked up Bible verses on my phone and read them aloud to him. Surprisingly, hearing the words calmed my spirit and soothed my soul. This became a daily practice for the duration of his hospital stay. It kept me grounded and helped me stay positive during this trying ordeal. It was weeks before I stumbled upon Psalm 118:17 (NIV), "I will not die but live, and will proclaim what the Lord has done." That day, I dedicated this Bible verse to my son, and I continue to speak it over him even today.

TAKEAWAY

This experience imparted two fundamental lessons that continue to resonate deeply with me. Firstly, in the darkest of moments, faith in God can serve as a powerful guiding light that illuminates the path ahead. This truth became tangible when the hospital's "one parent at a time" policy enforced isolation during such a challenging period. My faith and the reassuring words of God were the pillars of strength and support that carried me through that solitary time.

Secondly, I learned firsthand the importance of healthcare practitioners demonstrating empathy and compassion when interacting with parents. I often think back to how the surgeon's approach and words could have crushed my spirit, leading to an emotional spiral. Fortunately, there were individuals like the head doctor who had established a rapport with me, offering much-needed support and balance during this trying period.

CHAPTER 8

RECOVERY AND HOSPITAL STAY

Post-Surgery

The days that followed my baby's CDH (congenital diaphragmatic hernia) surgery were emotionally wringing. The surgeon's warning that he was still not yet out of the woods was like a heavy burden, a constant weight on my heart. Every off sound from his incubator sent my heart racing as I rushed to the worst-case scenario. This wasn't like me; I'd always seen myself as positive. But in that hospital room, sterile and filled with the scent of antiseptics, it seemed to bring out the worst in me.

Each day, I struggled through my own physical exhaustion and postpartum condition to go sit by his bedside. Each incubator had a lone stool, which wasn't ergonomically suited to postpartum stresses. Yet, I felt paralyzed to move, even to grab a bite to eat, as I was afraid he would succumb to his condition if I weren't there. A part of me knew this wasn't entirely rational, but the steady beeping of monitors seemed to echo my anxious heartbeat. It was as if the entire world had paused, and we were suspended in a state of uncertainty.

Instinctively, Robert and I found ourselves settling into a routine of managing things. I took on the daytime shift sitting with our baby, while Robert shouldered the responsibility of the night shift after his classes. However, this arrangement began to take its toll on our marriage, leaving us with limited opportunities to spend time together as a couple and as a family.

As the insomnia induced by stress persisted, I frequently found myself awake in the encompassing darkness of the night, straining to discern the faint sounds of Robert's car approaching our driveway during the early morning hours. On the one hand, I could perceive his deliberate attempts to move quietly as he entered our bedroom, believing I was fast asleep. On the other hand, I remained wide awake, my body utterly still, unable to find the words to initiate a conversation about the ongoing challenges with our child's health.

Thankfully, Robert usually succumbed to sleep swiftly, and before long, his exhausted snores would fill the room. As I lay there in silent obscurity, I would release a long-held breath while engaging in a combination of prayer, worry, and daydreaming about the moment when our son would finally come home. The darkness seemed to conceal and amplify the emotions that swirled within me during those anxious nights.

Each morning, I would rise from my bed early, knowing I was about to embark on the same routine again. My first order of business was preparing breakfast for my children and ensuring they were ready for school on weekdays. Only then would I head to the hospital, where I would remain for the entirety of the day, returning home in the late evening.

Amidst this relentless cycle, my blood pressure stubbornly remained high, resistant to all attempts at lowering it. It was as though my own well-being was in a race against time, but I couldn't bring myself to prioritize it. After all, this was my baby. The love and concern for his well-being overshadowed any personal concerns, and so I pressed on, driven by an unyielding determination to be there for him every step of the way.

Little did I realize that I had slipped into survival mode. With my health steadily deteriorating, my mind seemed to operate on autopilot, unable to engage in deep reflection or effective planning. Each day became a battle to make it through without succumbing to the immense weight that bore down on me.

Despite our decision to enlist the assistance of a live-in sitter to handle the physical aspects of our older children's care and the housekeeping chores, it was emotional and spiritual support that I yearned for desperately. However, I struggled to connect with anyone, including Cathy and Dave, who had been there for us when we initially discovered Nathan's CDH.

During my time at the hospital, I rarely ventured far from his side, taking only brief breaks to grab a bite or refresh myself hastily. I wanted to ensure he wasn't left alone. I was so wrapped up in my own world of worry that I didn't register the presence of the other mothers whose babies shared the same space as my son.

But I couldn't help but notice and internalize the daily battles unfolding before my eyes. I had a front-row seat to the fight for survival, witnessing babies experiencing one crisis after another multiple times throughout the day. These experiences were so jarring that each morning, I couldn't be certain I would see all the babies I had left there the night before. It chipped away at my very soul when I arrived to find a new baby in one of the other two incubators and was told that the previous occupant had passed away during the night. This heightened my worry and fear that my son could be next. As a result, leaving him to go home each night was excruciating, as I feared it might be the last time I would see him.

Once I was home, I longed for the moment when my children would settle into their beds for the night; only then could I immerse myself in the serene and comforting embrace of darkness. But as I lay in bed, I felt expectant, dreading what might be unfolding for my son at the hospital. Often, the phone's shrill ring would send a chill down my spine, causing my heart to race. I braced myself for the unimaginable news—that dreaded call from the hospital informing me of my son's passing. Yet, time and time again, it turned out to be a concerned friend or loved one on the other end reaching out for an update.

Moreover, I also found that when I spoke with extended family members or friends, my overpowering grief robbed me of my voice. For the first time in my life, I couldn't find words to express my feelings or even coherently explain what was happening with my son. Consequently, these well-intentioned calls often felt like an intrusion. I felt adrift, unsure of how to participate in life at that point. Every inquiry pushed me deeper into the abyss of despair, serving as a poignant reminder of the fragility and uncertainty that overshadowed our lives.

THE LONG WAIT

The waiting was unbearable. Day by day, after the surgery, my son's condition showed no signs of improvement. He lay in the incubator, his eyes closed, seemingly disconnected from the world around him. Uncertain of what more I could do, I turned to the Bible for consolation. A few days later, as I read aloud, a subtle movement caught my attention—a slight tilt of his head toward the sound of my voice. That was the moment when I first realized he was actually listening, forming a connection with my voice. This discovery filled me with immense hope and determination. From that day on, I made it a point to bring my Bible to the hospital with me each day.

During one of those reading sessions, I stumbled upon the very words that had been sent to me repeatedly during his surgery: "I will not die but live, and will proclaim what the Lord has done." [11] It struck me that this was an actual Bible verse and that it was personalized for my son. As I reflected on those powerful words, their significance became crystal clear. These words weren't sent to me by a mere coincidence; it was a divine message, a direct and intentional communication from God's heart to me and my son. This revelation strengthened my belief and made me hopeful that my son would overcome his challenges.

Despite this significant breakthrough, moments of agony still punctuated my days as I witnessed the delicate dance for life in the NICU. The isolation, the inability to have Robert or another family member with me, only added to the mounting frustration that was becoming increasingly difficult to bear. Each day felt like an emotional rollercoaster, a mix of hope and despair, as I traversed the challenges of my son's journey to recovery alone.

Amidst the prevailing darkness, a bright light emerged in the form of Dr. Sharon Smiles, a final-year resident pediatrician assigned to my son's case. The first time I met her, I was sitting

---

11 Psalm 118:17 (NIV)

with my son, feeling despondent when she entered the unit. Her presence was like a bright ray of sunshine. Her energy radiated, her passion for her craft, her warm smile, and her compassionate listening made me feel genuinely respected and heard. Unlike the surgeon, she didn't speak down to me or use medical jargon that left me confused. In fact, on several occasions when she was present with the surgeon, she took the initiative to simplify medical terminology and check in with me to ensure I was coping well emotionally.

One day, she asked me how I was holding up. At first, I gave the typical response, claiming that I was fine. But it was clear that she saw through that facade. Sensing my struggle, she then inquired about how I was coping with the stress of the situation. I hesitated for a moment and admitted that I was praying. My voice trailed off, and I felt a bit self-conscious, fearing that she, as a medical doctor grounded in the hard sciences, might view my prayers as trivial or irrational. To my surprise, she responded with a bright smile, saying, "Good, for I am praying for your son too." In that instant, I felt an extraordinary connection with her.

Dr. Smiles swiftly became the MVP[12] medically, someone I trusted and whose perspective mattered. She drew out my voice and constantly encouraged me to ask questions. She had remarkable patience and empathy even when I clumsily worded a question or concern. Instead of making me feel small, she artfully rephrased my inquiries before providing the information I needed. This helped to build my knowledge and confidence in speaking with my baby's healthcare team.

Another remarkable quality that she brought to our experience is that whenever "Dr. Doom" delivered disheartening up-

12 Most valuable player

dates, Dr. Smiles had a way of summarizing the information in a more positive light. For instance, when Dr. Doom would say, "We don't see any improvement in your son's health," Dr. Smiles would reframe it by saying, "As the doctor mentioned, your son is holding his own. Given what he's been through, it's expected that his body would need time to heal." Her reassuring words acted as a gentle stream of support, continuously replenishing our well of strength and hope during the most challenging moments.

In addition to her exceptional qualities, Dr. Smiles firmly believed in the transformative power of prayer. She consistently uplifted my spirits, encouraging me to maintain my faith and persevere in prayer. She would ensure I noticed the subtle indications of progress in his condition, underscoring the significance of these hopeful signs. I vividly recall a particular instance when she candidly shared that the medical team had done nothing different that could explain the improvements. She affirmed, "Prayer works. Keep praying, Mom."

THE HILLS AND VALLEYS

But as the days progressed, I discovered that the road to healing is not a straight path but a winding journey filled with hills, valleys, and plains. There were moments when hopeful signs suggested my son was making progress, but then, in the blink of an eye, he would suddenly experience a decline. This unpredictability filled me with uncertainty and enveloped his odds of survival in a shroud of darkness.

One of the darkest moments following the surgery unfolded on the ninth day post-operation. I was too weak and ill to make it to the hospital that day, so I took the day off. As I stepped into the NICU the next day, a nurse's sudden exclamation caught me completely off guard. "There she is, thank God," she urgently exclaimed, her eyes filled with deep concern. Her tone and expression instantly awakened the ever-present fear that had been lurking in the shadows. *Did something happen to my son?* The dread of losing him tightened its grip on my heart.

My mind swirled with worry as I was swiftly escorted into the neonatologist's[13] office. She wasted no time in coming to the heart of the matter. She explained that they had been trying to reach me for the past two days because my son had developed a high fever the evening after I left the hospital. Subsequent tests confirmed a severe case of jaundice.

The doctor paused, allowing the gravity of the situation to take hold, and then inquired if I was familiar with newborn jaundice. With a nod, I informed her that my previous children had also experienced newborn jaundice, which usually resolved with sunlight exposure after a few days. However, the doctor went on to explain that this particular case of jaundice was different. Because it occurred nine days after birth and six days after surgery, its onset may indicate a potential post-surgery complication.

She went on to explain that jaundice occurs when there is an accumulation of bilirubin, a substance produced during the breakdown of old red blood cells, in the bloodstream and tissues. The liver plays a vital role in breaking down bilirubin and facilitating its elimination through sweat, urine, and stools. However, any disruption in the process of bilirubin movement from the blood to the liver and its subsequent elimination from the body can result in jaundice[14].

---

13 Neonatologists are pediatricians in the NICU with specialized training in the care of critically ill newborns, particularly those born prematurely or with complex medical conditions.

14 Praveen Kumar Chandrasekharan, Munmun Rawat, Rajeshwari Madappa, David H. Rothstein, and Satyan Lakshminrusimha, "Congenital Diaphragmatic hernia—a review," Maternal

"The problem is," she began, her voice trailing off momentarily, "because your son's jaundice appeared so long after birth, we believe it is directly linked to his CDH condition and surgery. We know that these have impacted his body's ability to process and eliminate bilirubin effectively." She paused and said, "Two nights ago, during the midnight round of blood works, we found his bilirubin count very high."

"How high is high?" I inquired.

"408," she responded.

"What should it be?" I asked.

"Zero," she responded.

I didn't know what to make of the information. But thankfully, she didn't stop there.

"That is why we were trying to contact you," she continued. "We wanted to discuss the treatment options: blood exchange transfusion or phototherapy. But we couldn't find whole blood compatible with him, nor did we think he would survive a transfusion. So, when we couldn't reach you, we went with the less invasive option—phototherapy."

She then smiled for the first time and continued, "He started responding quickly to the treatment. As of this morning, his bilirubin levels are down to negligible levels and decreasing."

Overwhelmed with gratitude, I thanked her before hastening to see my son.

As I entered the room, my eyes widened in horror at the sight that greeted me. The previously inserted IV line, which had been in my son's hand or foot, was now uncomfortably placed in his head. The image was deeply unsettling and distressing, raising immediate concerns for me. The nurse walked in at that moment, and seeing the expression on my face, she reassured me that due to the extended usage of IV fluids, the veins in my son's hands and legs had collapsed, necessitating this alternative placement. Her words, that the sight appeared worse than it actually was, offered a small measure of solace. However, it was hard for me to look at, so I went outside for some fresh air.

I was walking toward my minivan when a familiar voice, the very same that had guided me through pivotal moments of my journey, resounded in my mind. It posed some thought-provoking questions, "Why are you sitting on the fence, waiting to see if he would die? Why has he not been formally named? Why is his room at home not prepared for his arrival?"

As I contemplated the questions honestly, I realized that I had been caught in indecision, unsure of which path to take. Perhaps the surgeon's prognosis, with its fifty-fifty chance of survival, had kept me perched on that fence. I then realized that instead of moving by faith, I was waiting to see what fate had in store. Until that moment, even though we had chosen his name months before his birth, he was solely referred to as "Baby Ebanks" by the healthcare staff or merely "the baby" by our family and friends. It became clear that it was time to make a resolute decision to shape our narrative in the way I envisioned. It was time for me to take a proactive step. It was time to give him his name.

TAKEAWAY

This part of my journey was profoundly emotional. It took me time and healing to recognize this experience's value. Two key takeaways emerged:

First, I discovered the power of resilience and patience. Throughout my baby's recovery challenges, I unearthed a well-spring of resilience within me that I hadn't known existed. I also learned the importance of patience, understanding that healing is a gradual process, and hope can sustain us through uncertainty.

Secondly, this chapter marked the beginning of my education on the significance of advocacy and communication. Navigating the intricacies of the healthcare system, I encountered health-care practitioners who sometimes treated me as if I possessed their level of expertise or, conversely, as if I couldn't understand. However, Dr. Smiles empowered me as an advocate, facilitating clearer communication with medical professionals and involving me in vital decision-making for my son's care. Little did I know that these vital skills would reach far beyond the confines of the hospital, arming me to become a passionate advocate for both social justice and the boundless love of a parent in advancing the cause of children with disabilities.

CHAPTER 9

MOMENTS OF FAITH AND PURPOSE

His Name Is Nathan

What's in a name? Bestowing a name upon a child is a profoundly symbolic and culturally significant tradition that intricately weaves the tapestry of a child's identity within the fabric of their family, society, and the wider world. It is a decision that parents undertake with meticulous care and profound consideration, acutely aware of the enduring imprint it will leave on their child's life.

Yet, despite my awareness of the significance of naming, at twelve days old, I had still not yet given him or called him by his name. In my mind, he was still "the baby," and we had not gone through the process of naming him, even though we had chosen a name months before I delivered him. As for why I did this, I can't quite explain it, but until that point, referring to him simply as "the baby" had felt easier for me.

Moreover, since we had chosen his name, expecting him to be exceptionally gifted, I struggled to reconcile that expectation with the reality of what was unfolding. I wasn't even sure if he would survive, and this uncertainty left me feeling immobilized.

But everything changed on the day when he miraculously survived the bout of jaundice. It was then that I realized I needed to decide. I chose to believe in his survival and his future. With firm conviction, I called home and instructed the sitter to prepare his room for his arrival. She asked if he was coming home that day; I told her no, but he was coming soon.

Then I realized it was time to give him his name officially. So, I set out for the Birth and Records office, which was a bit of a walk from the NICU. However, I didn't mind because my conviction that he would survive this grew stronger with each step.

On my way to the office, I phoned my church and spoke to my pastor's secretary. I shared with her the true nature of our struggle, as until then, the church family had only known that my son was born. I requested prayer support for my son and our family.

The office was nearly empty when I arrived, with only one officer working behind the counter. I provided her my name and delivery date, and she swiftly pulled up our records. When she inquired about his given name, I answered with a slight tremor in my voice, "Nathan Kingsley." She asked me to repeat it, and this time, it emerged as a confident declaration: "His name is Nathan Kingsley Ebanks." It was the moment when everything shifted. The utterance of his name held profound significance, solidifying his presence as not only my son but also a precious gift from God.

IDENTITY AND INDIVIDUALITY

Although I didn't realize it then, giving my son his name and addressing him by it made the experience of him more humanizing in my thoughts, helping me recognize him as an individual—a significant shift for me. As I walked back to the NICU building, my phone rang. It was Pastor Pat, one of the senior pastors from my church, returning my call. He attentively listened as I poured out my heart, tears streaming down my face. During our conversation, I referred to my son by his name and noticed that he did too. As he prayed, he called Nathan by name, and I couldn't help but be uplifted by that simple act. For the first time, my son felt like a person, not just a sick baby.

Suddenly, during the prayer, Pastor Pat paused. He shared that as he was praying, he had a vision of Jesus cradling Nathan in the palm of His hand. He went on to say that this vision was a sign that my son would be all right and survive what he was going through. His reassuring words filled me with a renewed sense of hope. It was precisely the reassurance I needed to strengthen my belief that my son would indeed overcome the challenges before him.

After the call ended, I immediately called Robert. I was eager to share the uplifting news, and I could hear the relief in his voice. A beautiful song of hope resonated within my spirit as I hung up the phone, and it seemed to reverberate with every step I took, infusing a newfound lightness into my stride.

A sense of calm washed over me for the first time since my son's admission, easing the usual urgency to rush back to his side. Instead, I took a detour to explore the parents' lounge, a space I had heard about but hadn't had the chance to visit before.

It was there, in the parents' lounge, that a serendipitous encounter occurred—I met another mom.

A Lesson in Community Support

As I tentatively entered the lounge, which was just off the NICU entrance, I immediately noticed three women huddled together, engrossed in a deep conversation. I didn't recognize any of them, although it was unlikely that I would have, as I usually moved about with my focus straight ahead, rarely looking to the left or right.

With polite nods, they acknowledged my arrival before resuming their lively discussion. As I settled into my seat, I unintentionally found myself listening in. One voice, whom I will refer to as Mother #1, stood out as she shared intricate details of her baby's health condition.

According to her account, her son had been born with a congenital heart defect six months before. He had been transferred to the University Hospital of the West Indies (UHWI), where specialized medical care could be accessed. However, up to that point, he remained too fragile to undergo surgery. Consequently, Mother #1 had been making the journey to Kingston from a considerable distance for the past six months to be by her baby's side. Due to affordability, she had been sleeping in the parents' lounge on the very uncomfortable-looking sofa. It touched my heart.

Her story deeply moved me, especially when I learned that she had three young children at home, just like me. However, unlike me, she didn't have the support of a husband or partner, and there was no family she could call on. An elderly neighbor was looking after her children in her absence.

Mothers #2 and #3 also shared their stories, and while their situations weren't as dire as Mother #1's, they were equally compelling. They spoke of the devastation, heartbreak, and emotional struggles they were going through—common experiences that we all shared. This encounter with these mothers opened my eyes to the significance of community and the need for support for parents enduring such hardships. It saddened me to realize that this need wasn't acknowledged or addressed by the hospital. There were no support systems in place for parents like us. We were left on our own to cope with the challenges we faced concerning our children's health.

To my surprise, all three women shared that they had noticed me passing by each day and had wanted to reach out but thought I looked unapproachable. It was a moment of self-awareness as I recognized how my own struggles had unknowingly isolated me from others, even from the mother who shared the same space with me as I sat by my son.

After Mothers #2 and #3 left, Mother #1 and I fell into a comfortable silence. Unexpectedly, she asked if I was a Christian. Though I was surprised by the directness of her question, I told her I was. She laughed aloud, clapping her hands as she said she knew it. She mentioned something about how I carried myself and spoke. Then, she shared that she had started attending church during her pregnancy but hadn't returned due to her son's hospitalization. She expressed that she had wanted to surrender her life to Christ for some time, but the opportunity hadn't presented itself—until now. She asked if I could lead her in praying the sinner's prayer of repentance.

I was taken aback. I had not thought of myself in that role, believing it was the domain of pastors and ministers. Initially, I hesitated, but her earnestness compelled me to set aside my reservations. With a tinge of self-consciousness, I joined her in prayer, listening to her confession of her sins, repentance, and invitation for Christ to enter her heart and guide her life. It marked an unforgettable moment that moments of faith and purpose can still blossom amidst our shared suffering and challenges. I couldn't shake the feeling that our meeting had a deeper, spiritual significance beyond the medical reasons for my and her son's presence in the hospital at the same time.

As I prepared to bid her farewell, I felt a powerful urge stirred within me to offer her a gift. Our encounter left me feeling immensely blessed and uplifted, and her story touched my heart in a profound way. Yet, out of shyness, I hesitated. The thoughts that came to mind were to give her the Bible I always carried in my car and the money in my purse. While parting with the money didn't pose a significant challenge, the Bible held sentimental value as a cherished childhood gift from my mother. It contained precious notes, birthday blessings, prayers, and other treasured information. So, I brushed my thoughts aside, said goodbye, and went to see my son.

That evening marked the first night I left the hospital in good spirits. For the first time, my mind was not on my son or our circumstances but on Mother #1 and my prayers for her and her family.

TAKEAWAY

Although I didn't realize it then, bestowing my son with his name and addressing him by it within the hospital and during

110

conversations with others transformed his experience from being just a patient (baby Ebanks) to acknowledging his individuality. This act humanized the entire experience, both for him and our family. I want to think that even though he was still so young, it assisted him in understanding that he was not merely another medical case but a one-of-a-kind and cherished individual.

Second, I learned that having a strong support system rooted in faith, family, and community can make a significant difference in navigating the challenges of waiting and uncertainty. Such a network offers essential emotional, spiritual, and practical assistance, providing comfort, encouragement, and a sense of belonging during difficult times.

CHAPTER 10

CONNECTING THREADS OF HOPE AND SUPPORT

Trusting My Intuition: A Valuable Lesson

That weekend, the impact of meeting Mother #1 lingered with me. It symbolized a significant shift in my perspective. I had moved away from my constant preoccupation with Nathan and started to consider the experiences of other mothers who were going through similar challenges and in need of support.

Upon arriving at the NICU on Monday morning, I entered the parents' lounge with a sense of purpose, carrying the gifts that had been pressing on my heart since my initial encounter with Mother #1. However, she was nowhere to be seen. Her conspicuous absence persisted throughout the week, escalating the worry shared by both myself and the other mothers. We couldn't help but wonder what might have caused her uncharacteristic absence.

I prayed that everything was all right with her and her family.

As I entered the NICU the following week, I heard Mother #1 calling out to me. I was overjoyed to see her and felt a wave of relief. We embraced each other warmly and exchanged greetings like old friends. Unable to contain my curiosity, I inquired about her absence the previous week. She explained that she had exhausted all her funds to travel back home the day we initially met, which left her with no means to return to the hospital. It was only now that she had managed to secure the assistance she needed to come back.

Her words filled me with remorse as I understood why I had gotten the prompting the last time we were together to assist her with some money. Excusing myself, I hurried to my car to retrieve the Bible. Hastily, I placed the money from my purse into an envelope and rushed back to the lounge to present it to her alongside the Bible. I explained that I had felt the urge to do so the day we met. She was visibly moved as she accepted the gifts. Strangely, as grateful as she was for the money, her joy over the Bible was even more profound. She began dancing, explaining that she had been praying for a full Bible for over a year, having only owned a New Testament Bible until now. She saw the gift as a divine answer to her prayers and an affirmation that God was indeed listening. As she turned to look into my eyes, her words held a profound weight, "Mommy Ebanks, I realize we are here because our babies are sick. But I feel thankful that we are here. Because if it weren't for our babies, we probably would never have met, and meeting you has changed my life more than you can ever understand. Thank you for taking the chance to stop in this room and talk with me. Thank you for your support and help. It goes to show everything is connected to everything."

Her heartfelt gratitude and reflection on the connection between our paths touched me deeply. It was humbling to realize how a moment and an act that seemed small to me could be huge for another. Her situation also sparked gratitude in my heart as I realized that as bad as I thought I had things, others had it worse. Indeed, it underscored the unexpected ways life weaves its tapestry of connections. I also realized that embracing our community and reaching out can be a powerful source of support, understanding, and hope amidst the trials we face. These connections forged during challenging times can be a lifeline to ourselves or someone else, offering strength and comfort and affirming that we are not alone in our struggles.

After saying our goodbyes, we went our separate ways. As I walked away, a sense of peace enveloped me, a deep feeling of fulfillment. It was instinctual, knowing we'd never meet again, yet I embraced it, carrying the conviction that my presence there had indeed served a purpose. I also sensed that my son's time at the hospital was nearing its end.

A JOURNEY NEARING ITS END

After my visit with Mother #1, I felt renewed hope as I headed to see Nathan again. However, when I reached the incubator room, I was surprised to find a new baby in his stead. Somehow, I wasn't alarmed, as deep down, I had a sense that my son was okay. A trace of anxiety lingered as I stepped out and spotted a nurse hurrying toward me. I asked her about my son's location and why there was another baby in his incubator. She quickly reassured me, explaining that Nathan was making excellent progress. He had been taken off extensive support overnight and was now resting in a cot in the outer room, a clear and reassuring indicator of his improving condition. She explained that they had intended to surprise me upon my arrival, but unfortunately, they missed me when I first entered.

She gently guided me back to the center of the room, and I saw my son there. I wouldn't have recognized him at first glance without the bandages and tubes obscuring him. It was the first time I could see his entire face, revealing my child's features to me for the first time, and he was twenty-one days old. He still needed oxygen support, which was provided by a tiny Pooh Bear mask and a small portable tank.

The moment filled me with a whirlwind of emotions. I felt an overwhelming sense of relief and pure joy at finally being able to see my child's face, and tears of happiness welled up in my eyes. It was a moment of wonder and awe as I took in every detail of his delicate features for the very first time. Emotionally, it was intense, marking a significant milestone in our journey together and giving me hope for his continued progress. My heart was brimming with love, gratitude, and an indescribable connection with my child.

He was also dressed in the onesie, booties, and adorable cap I had brought to the hospital on his birthday. In those clothes, he looked like an entirely different child. He was picture-perfect, and that moment is etched into my mind forever. Whenever life gets tough for him, I often revisit that cherished memory of his strength as an overcomer.

That day, I accomplished numerous first-time milestones: holding him, kissing him, and cuddling him. It marked the first time I could breastfeed him, change his diaper, and dress him. It all felt surreal, and I was filled with gratitude that he was among the survivors, defying the odds that had been stacked against him since before birth. As I held him, I offered up prayers for the other babies in the unit and their families. I prayed for all the parents who had lost their children's battles in the weeks we spent there, hoping they would find strength and healing in their journeys.

After that day, everything seemed to move rapidly. The nurses arranged for him to meet his siblings, oxygen tank and all. My eyes welled up with tears as I witnessed them showering him with hugs and kisses. They expressed their love for him, eagerly sharing how they couldn't wait for him to come home. A smile spread across my face as Jordanne, ever curious, asked where her baby brother's hair was. It was the first time I realized that he was completely bald—no hair on his head, eyebrows, or lashes. The sight of my children coming together, filled with love and excitement, was a heartwarming moment that I will forever cherish.

Two days later, I arrived at the hospital and once again passed Nathan on the way in. They had moved him closer to the entrance, and the oxygen mask was gone. Admittedly, I wasn't so confident then, as I worried about whether they should be doing that. That was when the what-ifs first appeared. *What if he needs oxygen, and they didn't notice? What if...*

Finally, the long-awaited moment arrived—the day Nathan was discharged. As he underwent his final checks with the surgeon (Dr. Doom), I couldn't help but capture a photo of them together. She asked why I had taken the picture. I shared my belief that a young man would one day approach her and say, "I know you. You are the doctor who saved my life." However, she responded by saying, "This child is still not out of the woods. He might not even survive infancy or childhood."

I was so elated that he was finally coming home that not even her poorly worded response fazed me. I thanked her for her service and confidently stated that my son would live and not die, proclaiming the glory of God. She smiled at my response, which was the first glimpse of humanity I had seen in her over the duration of his hospitalization. After a few post-operation check-ups with her, we walked out of the hospital with our baby. It was May 28, 2004, twenty-four days after he was born.

As I basked in the sight of my son, peacefully asleep in his infant seat, I believed that the worst was behind us. After all we had endured, I couldn't imagine what could surpass those challenges. We saw Dr. Doom twice after that in the coming weeks for wound checkups and bandage changes. After that, he was discharged to the outpatient services. We never saw her again.

Little did I realize that this only marked the end of one chapter and the beginning of another.

TAKEAWAY

The takeaway from the chapter "Connecting Threads of Hope and Support" is deeply significant for me. First, my connection with the other mothers, particularly Mother #1, gave me the precious gift of perspective, which helped me realize that I had the financial means and family support to aid my son and carry us through this crisis. I resided in Kingston, blessed with a beautiful home and motor vehicles that facilitated my journeys to and from the hospital. The mere thought of it being otherwise, where I lacked these resources like some of the mothers I had the privilege of meeting, sent shudders down my spine. However, this stark contrast compelled me to shift my perspective toward gratitude for what I did possess rather than dwelling on what I lacked.

Second, I learned to see purpose in everything because as I extended my hand to help another, it seemed as though a greater plan was at work, contributing to my son's healing journey. While I acknowledge the oversimplification of this perspective, it offered me comfort and strength during that challenging period. It underscored the intricate interconnectedness of our life experiences and highlighted the potential for positive transformation when we take the time to help others, regardless of the challenges we may be facing ourselves.

CHAPTER 11

THROUGH THE MAZE OF UNCERTAINTY: OUR JOURNEY TO DIAGNOSIS

Here We Go Again!

Nathan received a warm welcome when we arrived home. Our extended family and close friends had gathered to greet us, making it a joyous and celebratory occasion. His siblings were overflowing with excitement, eager to hold him. Amidst the warmth of the moment, I couldn't help but recall the wise words of a compassionate nurse who had spent a significant amount of time with Nathan during his hospitalization. Before we departed, she shared invaluable advice with a kind and knowing smile, which left a lasting impression on me.

She had dedicated much of her career to neonatal care in En-gland and worked with children with congenital diaphragmatic hernia (CDH). She explained that Nathan would be medically fragile for quite some time, but we mustn't treat him as broken. Instead, she urged us to embrace the presence of his siblings, explaining that they were the greatest gift we could offer him. She cautioned against shielding him from them and encouraged us to involve them in his life from the moment he was home. Even though they were young, she advised us to teach them how to assist us in caring for their little brother. Furthermore, she stressed the importance of allowing them to play and interact with him, recognizing that their love and companionship would foster an unbreakable bond and help normalize his life.

The nurse's words resonated deeply, influencing how I approached integrating Nathan into our family. Taking her advice to heart, I carefully arranged pillows so that each sibling could have a moment to hold him. It was tough to separate them from him that night, so they slept in his room. They were so attached and concerned that we kept them home from school for a few days, as they feared he wouldn't be there when they returned home. Fortunately, their understanding teachers granted them the time they needed.

But, just like our family and friends, we believed that our challenging journey had come to an end. Unfortunately, we were never informed that Nathan's experiences, such as surgery, prolonged oxygen usage, and developing jaundice, put him at a high risk for developmental delays. We were never referred to early intervention and were ill-prepared to recognize any early warning signs of these delays. In fact, when these signs initially emerged, we were unaware of their significance, and it turned out that even the doctors in the post-surgery outpatient department were in the same boat.

RED FLAGS AND EARLY WARNING SIGNS

I dutifully took Nathan for post-surgery follow-ups twice per week for several weeks. I was feeling increasingly ill, but despite the mounting difficulties, I persevered silently, harboring a deep-seated fear that acknowledging my illness to anyone would lead to my own hospitalization. The thought of being away from my recovering baby filled me with dread. Except for Robert, I kept my worsening condition carefully concealed.

However, the persistent shortness of breath, loss of appetite, and excruciating headaches eventually compelled me to seek medical attention. Concerned, I made an appointment with my doctor. My worst fears were confirmed after a series of tests—I had postpartum eclampsia[15]. My blood pressure had reached dangerously high levels, and the presence of all these symptoms—severe headaches, blurry vision, abdominal pain, and nausea—were clear warning signs. However, I was unaware of their significance at the time.

My treatment plan involved managing my high blood pressure with medication, getting ample rest, staying well-hydrated, and adhering to a carefully monitored diet. Additionally, I was prescribed pain medication to alleviate my persistent headaches.

However, it became a delicate balancing act as I navigated my own health challenges while simultaneously caring for the needs of Nathan and his siblings. The responsibilities felt overwhelming, and I sometimes questioned whether I would make

---

15 Postpartum eclampsia is a rare but serious medical condition that can occur in some women after childbirth. It is a severe complication of preeclampsia, a condition that typically occurs during pregnancy and is characterized by high blood pressure (hypertension) and damage to organs such as the liver and kidneys. Eclampsia is essentially the progression of preeclampsia to a more severe and life-threatening stage.

it through the night to see a new day. The burden of stress and worries intensified my insomnia, leaving me restless throughout the night.

As my own health hung in the balance, we started to notice concerning developments in Nathan's growth and development. Initially, I had assumed that he would gradually improve as the weeks went by, so I wasn't actively looking for signs of trouble, even though they were becoming increasingly evident. It took me some time to recognize these signs in hindsight. Even if I had been more vigilant, I wouldn't have grasped the complete significance of these signs because developmental delays had never been discussed as a potential concern, and I had no prior knowledge of what they entailed.

TRUSTING MY GUT: A LESSON IN MATERNAL INSTINCTS

Deep within me, I held an intuition that something was amiss with my baby's development. At eight weeks old, he still responded much like a newborn, struggling with feeding, frequently vomiting after meals, and battling recurrent episodes of acute constipation, which proved challenging to alleviate even with enemas.

My concerns deepened as I noticed his difficulty focusing his eyes on objects right before him. Tummy time on his activity mat was a struggle, and he couldn't muster the strength to roll over or change positions. At three months, my attempt to prop him up for a sitting position revealed a lack of muscle tone reminiscent of a fragile newborn. Holding him felt different from the typical sensation of cradling a person. His body lacked muscle tone, rendering it exceptionally soft and relaxed as if he might slip from my grasp at any moment. This stunted development only intensified my concerns and left me feeling utterly helpless.

His cry, or more accurately, the absence of it, was yet another source of worry. I would watch as silent tears streamed down his face, devoid of any sound. It was a heart-wrenching sight. I later discovered that this was a lasting effect of his prolonged intubation during his hospital stay. It would be several months before he began to make any vocal sounds, and it took another two years before he developed the lung strength to produce loud sounds.

I meticulously documented my observations and brought them to the post-surgery clinic visits, hoping for clarity and reassurance. However, when I raised these concerns, seeking guidance, the doctor would dismiss them with casual remarks, suggesting that these issues were temporary and that he would eventually "grow out of them." But I knew deep down that something was profoundly wrong.

As Nathan ended his fourth month and the developmental delays became increasingly pronounced, I realized it was time to seek a second, or even a third, opinion. I felt completely out of my depth because all my other children had consistently met or exceeded their developmental milestones. I had always taken pride in their achievements, considering them above average. Consequently, the thought never crossed my mind to contemplate the significance of a child experiencing delays in their developmental milestones or the complexities of child development.

Lacking the necessary guidance, I remained unaware that these delays could be indicative of underlying conditions or disabilities that persist throughout a person's life, necessitating ongoing management and support. None of this crucial information had been discussed with me during Nathan's hospitalization or at the post-surgery clinic.

But my own red flags persisted, pushing me to the brink. One night, as I lay in bed, it felt like my organs were shutting down. While my children and husband peacefully slept, I struggled with the fear of dying. I didn't know if it was real or imagined, but I knew I could not continue like that. So, I awakened Robert, told him how I felt, and asked him to keep watch over me for the night. Then I prayed, "Dear Lord, I feel like my life is slipping away. Yet, I recall Your promise at the start of my pregnancy that Nathan is a gift from You. While I know You can use another to raise him, I feel that our purposes are intertwined. Therefore, I am asking You to spare my life so that I may live to raise my son and fulfill Your plans for us. Grant me the gift of rest tonight. Amen."

After my prayer, exhaustion overcame me, and I fell into a deep sleep. I slept for fourteen hours, succumbing to the weariness accumulated throughout my challenging journey. When I awoke the next day, the symptoms of the night before had decreased. I was on the mend. However, that was the night Robert's struggle with insomnia started. It would be years before he learned to manage it.

With my own health improving, my determination to find answers for my son was reignited. Frustrated by the limited attention my concerns had received from the doctors at the post-surgery clinic, after discussing it with Robert, we agreed that it was time to take Nathan to another doctor. I made an appointment with Dr. Houston, one of the pediatricians who saw my other children.

TAKEAWAY

This experience has taught me the significant role parents, particularly maternal instincts, play in early diagnosis and intervention. Even when I was unwell myself, I had an intuition that something wasn't right with my son's development. In my role as his primary caregiver, I never left his side, and I discovered that this held importance, for while I may not have possessed medical expertise, my gut instincts were remarkably accurate. Only years later, when I became involved in advocacy, I discovered that in Jamaica, children were often diagnosed much later, typically between eighteen months and three years old. This delay meant that valuable time for early intervention was lost.

Second, I learned that our keen observations and insights as parents are invaluable to healthcare professionals and therapists, providing essential insights during the evaluation and treatment processes. We are central in the decision-making process, offering a unique perspective that aids practitioners in taking into account our family dynamics and the broader context that shapes our child's development. Thus, our voices are essential in shaping the best possible interventions and support for our children.

CHAPTER 12

THE ROAD TO DIAGNOSIS: FITTING TOGETHER THE PIECES OF THE PUZZLE

The First Appointment

I was nervous when I took Nathan to his first appointment with Dr. Houston. I sensed something was amiss, yet I held onto the hope that it wouldn't turn out to be anything too serious. Our decision to bring Nathan to the same pediatric clinic where his siblings received care was reassuring. Dr. Houston, whom I had a good rapport with, happened to be available. Little did I know, this choice to seek another professional opinion marked the initial stride toward uncovering a diagnosis.

As I was sitting in the waiting room, my mind raced with many questions and uncertainties. Would today be the day we finally uncovered what had been causing our sweet Nathan's developmental delays and unique challenges? The weight of the unknown bore me down, making the wait to see the doctor feel like an eternity.

Dr. Houston's warm smile greeted us as we entered his office, instantly putting me at ease. He knew us well, having cared for our other children, but this time was different. This time, we needed answers.

I could tell right away that Dr. Houston was deeply concerned about Nathan's presentation. He displayed a level of thoroughness that put my worries at ease. He meticulously reviewed our medical records and conducted a comprehensive examination of Nathan. To my relief, Dr. Houston acknowledged my observation that Nathan was indeed experiencing delays in all his developmental milestones, with the exception of his height. His words reassured me, confirming that my proactive approach in seeking answers had been the right course of action. Finally, finding a doctor who shared our perspective on Nathan's development reinforced our belief that we were making the right strides in securing the help he needed. Dr. Houston proposed a series of tests and devised a well-structured plan to closely monitor specific developmental milestones over the course of two months. He also took the time to ensure I understood the milestones and their significance—how they should naturally manifest and why they played a crucial role in assessing Nathan's progress.

Together, we committed to a schedule of biweekly appointments, each one a stepping stone on this uncertain path. It was the beginning of a journey we had not anticipated, a journey that would demand patience, resilience, and unyielding hope.

DIAGNOSTIC EVALUATION

Something extraordinary and seemingly serendipitous occurred the evening before Nathan's final monitoring appointment with Dr. Houton. By chance, I stumbled upon a documentary on television that focused on the life of a mother who had made the challenging choice to leave her job to provide dedicated care for her son. The child caught my attention. He was around eight and sat in a specialized wheelchair that resembled a large stroller. As the mother shared their story, she explained that her son had received a diagnosis of cerebral palsy, a disability that significantly impacted their lives. She described how this diagnosis had transformed their daily routines, as her son required assistance with everyday living activities such as eating, bathing, and using the bathroom.

I found myself captivated by her story, a sudden and undeniable awareness that my son shared the same condition as her son. It was my first encounter with this particular diagnosis, almost as if it were a divine foreshadowing, getting me ready for the impending appointment with Dr. Houston the very next day.

The Saturday morning dawned bright and beautiful. Robert stayed home with our other children, and I took Nathan to the appointment. As we stepped into Dr. Houston's office that Saturday morning, I couldn't shake the feeling that our lives were teetering on the edge of a significant turning point. Dr. Houston welcomed us warmly and initiated the assessment of the milestones we had painstakingly monitored.

As he completed the assessment, he leaned back in his chair, making direct eye contact with me, signaling that an important conversation would occur. "I understand that this conversation is undoubtedly difficult for you," he said. "As you know, we have closely monitored Nathan's development over the past two months. Regrettably, he continues to exhibit global developmental delay at six months old, consistent with cerebral palsy. To better understand his condition, I would like to refer him to a neurologist for further assessment and evaluation. This step will aid us in obtaining an official diagnosis for him, enabling us to delve deeper into the specific nature of his condition. This understanding is of utmost importance as it will allow us to create a comprehensive care plan tailored to his unique and specific needs. After all he has been through, I am sorry to be the bearer of such bad news. But please know that I am committed to offering as much information and assistance as possible."

As I exited the doctor's office that day, clutching the referral in my hand and pushing Nathan's stroller with the other, I experienced a strange mix of emotions. Numbness enveloped me, yet there was also a sense of relief. The news served as confirmation that I wasn't merely imagining things—there truly was something significant amiss in my baby's development.

As I drove us home, my emotions swung between shock at the weight of the diagnosis and simmering anger. I realized that precious months had been wasted, futilely expressing my concerns to the doctor at the outpatient surgery clinic. If only they had taken me seriously, my baby could have received the necessary help and support he needed.

I needed some time alone to process everything. I arrived home but desired solitude with my thoughts. I asked Robert to come and take care of Nathan, and once he had him, I drove off to have some space for myself. A whirlwind of questions and uncertainties flooded my mind. *What exactly was cerebral palsy? Is it contagious? How would it shape my son's life, as well as the lives of myself and my family? Did I have the strength for this? Is it permanent or temporary? Is there a cure? Can it be fixed? Healed? Did I do something wrong to cause this condition? Would it put my son's life in jeopardy?*

As I continued driving, I longed for someone to assure me that it was all just a dream or a misunderstanding. This was not the life I had envisioned for my precious "gift from God." Where was the blessing in all he had been through? Gradually, a sense of stillness settled in, and memories of Nathan's incredible resilience and the miraculous journey he had been on flooded my mind.

The miles stretched on, and I lost track of time, lost in deep reflection. However, amidst the uncertainty, clarity slowly began to emerge. Regardless of the challenges that lay ahead with the diagnosis, one truth remained unwavering—I loved my son unconditionally. Though I didn't fully grasp how the diagnosis would impact us, I knew that my focus must be on Nathan and his well-being. I understood that I would need to learn and understand my role in supporting him through this journey.

I recalled a poignant prayer I had made that fateful night when I thought I was dying. I had made a promise to my son before God to be his advocate, to help him unlock his unique potential and the gifts he carried within him. I was determined to support him in fulfilling his purpose in the world.

With newfound clarity, renewed commitment, and unwavering determination, I knew it was time to head home and have a heart-to-heart conversation with Robert. After all, this was only the beginning of our journey with the diagnosis.

TAKEAWAY

I'm grateful that we recognized the importance of seeking professional help, following our instincts, and choosing the right healthcare professional in this aspect of the journey. Many of the families I've encountered over the years took different paths. Some, who are believers, chose to spiritualize the condition and didn't seek professional support. As a result, even after years, they still didn't fully understand the disability and what was required to help their child.

I'm grateful that we understood the intricate interplay between the spiritual and medical realms at this integral phase of our journey. This enabled us to recognize that God often works through the dedicated professionals in the healthcare field. These doctors and healthcare providers are pivotal in helping diagnose, treat, and prevent illnesses, all while offering vital support for our health and well-being. Their primary mission of enhancing the quality of life for individuals and entire communities, easing suffering, and fostering overall well-being makes them incredible allies in our journey—both toward diagnosis and in raising a child with a disability.

CHAPTER 13

UNDERSTANDING THE DIAGNOSIS: MOVING BEYOND PUZZLE PIECES

God's Sovereignty and Purpose in Diagnosis

We had our first meeting with the neurologist when Nathan was seven months old. He was an imposing man, even though his stature was frail. He was well-known and respected in the field, and I was hopeful for what his services would deliver. I didn't understand what the disability meant, and the day we met with him, I was expectant for a cure.

The neurologist, unfortunately, didn't offer much information during that crucial meeting. Instead, he directed us to undergo a battery of tests, one of which was an MRI. Looking back now, the irony of this situation strikes me because the MRI necessitates complete stillness during its duration, which posed a significant challenge for Nathan, given his movement disorder due to cerebral palsy. Nevertheless, we were determined to get through it and took Nathan for the test, during which he needed to be sedated. All these expenses, including the doctors' visits, the test cost, and sedation, came directly out of our pockets.

The day we received the formal diagnosis in January 2005 is etched indelibly in my mind, a fateful memory. After thoroughly reviewing the test results, the neurologist delivered the solemn news that our son Nathan had athetoid dyskinetic cerebral palsy. He also pointed out that the brain scan had revealed swelling in Nathan's brain. Rather than offering guidance to help us understand the significance of these findings and the potential paths forward, the doctor chose to convey a disheartening message: that with this diagnosis, no therapy or treatment could make a difference, and we needed to come to terms with the fact that our son would face permanent disability. Though Nathan was only nine months old at the time, he went on to say that he would never walk, talk, function independently, attend a "normal" school, and no matter how much money we might invest, these circumstances would remain unchanged.

Despite the disheartening news, I reached for my notebook in my handbag and began diligently jotting down everything the doctor said. It appeared that he misunderstood my actions, possibly thinking that I was being indifferent, maybe assuming that we should be falling apart by the grim diagnosis. He expressed concern, telling me that I wasn't taking the information seriously.

I reassured him that I was taking it very seriously. But I also understood that his extensive experience in his field might have led him to believe that giving us a "reality check" was the right course of action. I pointed out that no one could truly predict my son's future outcomes with certainty and that, ultimately, it was in God's hands. I mentioned that I was taking detailed notes to guide my prayers on the matter. This response seemed to surprise him and catch him off guard.

After we left the appointment, I couldn't help but reflect on what I would have liked to say to him. I wanted him to understand that my intention wasn't to be disrespectful but to convey my sense that, as parents, we deserved respect, compassion, and empathy on this difficult journey. While this was another patient case for him, it was my child, whom I had carried in my body for nine months. Therefore, it was crucial that he left me with a measure of hope. I firmly believed that hope was what would empower me to draw strength and inspire resilience in the journey of raising this child. Consequently, I couldn't accept his fatalistic perspective as the last word.

Whenever I've shared this story, I often describe that consultation as the "never-never-ever meeting" because, in essence, that was all we took away from it. At that time, I also left the appointment believing cerebral palsy (CP) spelled a death sentence for my son. It was at that point that I began mentally preparing for the worst. But that night, in the privacy of my bedroom, I poured my heart out to God. Letting the tears flow unabatedly, I wept for my son and his future. I presented the lab report about the swelling on his brain, got down on my knees, and prayed a simple prayer, "God, this is what man says. What do You say?" Those were the only words I could find for my prayers that night, but I was expectant.

We repeated the brain scan a month later, and this time, the report indicated that the results were unremarkable. There was no evidence of swelling, and the scan did not reveal any noteworthy or abnormal features in his brain. What was once present had now disappeared. This marked a significant triumph for Robert and me, reaffirming our belief that God was indeed attentive to our prayers.

As the months passed, the true extent of the condition became increasingly evident. The challenges associated with dyskinetic athetoid cerebral palsy (CP) began manifesting more prominently in his everyday life. Due to persistent, involuntary movements, simple actions such as reaching for objects, sitting up, or feeding were difficult for him. Furthermore, communication challenges, or the lack thereof, increased, making it difficult for us to understand his needs and emotions. For instance, he didn't cry when he was hungry, sleepy, experiencing discomfort like needing a diaper change, feeling overstimulated, or even when he was sick. This presented us with the challenge of establishing a vigilant schedule and ensuring that someone was always with him to consistently meet these essential needs.

In addition to contending with motor and communication challenges, it became evident that developmental milestones such as crawling, walking, and speaking were not unfolding naturally. This situation necessitated intensive therapy. Unfortunately, besides physical therapy (PT), the other essential services were not readily accessible. Even if they were, affordability posed a significant hurdle as there was no available social support to help cover the costs of this necessary care.

The presence of spasticity and muscle tightness further intensified his discomfort, introducing an additional layer of complexity into our daily lives. To effectively cope with the challenges of his physical care, we had to enlist the assistance of his siblings, as it would have been too much for Robert and me to manage on our own. The experience was physically, mentally, and emotionally draining and exhausting for all of us. It robbed me of my joy.

But even as I struggled through the impact of the diagnosis, one comforting truth that kept me grounded was my faith in God's sovereignty. As Christians, Robert and I firmly believe that nothing occurs by chance in our lives; every circumstance, even a diagnosis as complex as our son's cerebral palsy, serves a divine purpose ordained by our heavenly Father. In the long days of caring for Nathan's daily needs, I found assurance in knowing that God's sovereign hand was at work even when I couldn't see it or understand it, especially through the chaotic moments of our new life.

I even drew comfort reflecting on biblical examples where God consistently demonstrated His sovereignty in the face of adversity and diagnoses. Take the story of Job, a man who faced unimaginable suffering and loss. Through his trials, Job's unwavering faith in God's sovereignty prevailed, and in the end, God restored his fortunes manifold. Similarly, in John 9, we encounter the account of a man born blind. Jesus used this man's condition not as a result of sin but as an opportunity to demonstrate God's power and reveal His glory. These stories reminded me during those long, dark moments of care and searching for answers that God can work through our situations to display His glory and reveal His plan.

SHIFTING PERSPECTIVES AND BREAKING STEREOTYPES

Accepting the cerebral palsy diagnosis was very challenging. For a while, I struggled to understand what the condition meant practically. *What was I required to do as a mother? How do I help my son's development? What does this mean for my life? My ca-reer?* For a period, I interpreted the disability through a spiritual lens, fervently believing that miraculous healing, a cure, or a fix was the only way to fulfill the divine promise associated with my child. Simultaneously, I pursued medical avenues for potential solutions. Due to my limited understanding of how the disability affected Nathan's growth and development, I grew increasingly frustrated and disheartened when these solutions failed to produce the desired change for him.

I diligently adhered to a schedule of quarterly visits to the neurologist, all in the hope that these appointments would catalyze positive improvements in my son's condition. Yet, it was disheartening to see his developmental delays remain unchanged. At each visit, the doctor primarily emphasized Nathan's limitations, highlighting his lack of progress in both gross motor skills, such as rolling over and sitting up, and fine motor skills, including grasping objects, hand-eye coordination, and finger dexterity, and I diligently recorded copious notes. Given that I was already aware of Nathan's limitations, I eagerly anticipated discussions about the areas in which he was progressing on schedule. I hoped for some glimmer of hope that not all was lost. However, these appointments consistently concluded without the doctor providing insights or guidance on supporting Nathan's development at home. Without fail, my shyness prevented me from pressing for further information, and I would leave those appointments with a profound sense of disappointment and sadness.

What made these appointments even more disheartening was the doctor's tendency to dismiss the developments we saw as positive. Instead, he often attributed them to mere ticks, symptoms of cerebral palsy, or even seizures (although Nathan had never been diagnosed with seizures). It seemed that no matter how age-appropriate behaviors such as learning to pinch others, brushing food off his tongue when he didn't like it, or closing his eyes when faced with exercise tasks he disliked, these actions were consistently attributed solely to his condition. As time went on, this intense preoccupation with his limitations clouded my perception of my son's true self and individuality. I momentarily lost sight of the wonderful child he was, becoming fixated solely on his limitations, unintentionally neglecting his other wonderful qualities and the aspects of his development that were progressing as expected. Sadly, during that period, every time I looked at my child, all I saw was only his disability.

As time went on, I started to question the purpose of these visits to the neurologist. We were paying a significant amount out of pocket, yet, aside from taking notes, the doctor never provided any useful information or addressed my questions to offer the much-needed clarity we sought. These routine visits strained my monthly household budget and left me feeling angry, frustrated, and deeply disappointed.

During this disheartening cycle, I found myself feeling completely adrift. It seemed as though my only option was to persist in my search for answers because, in my perspective, the alternative was simply giving up. Yet, giving up was never a realistic choice for me. I believed I owed it to my son to exhaust every possible avenue to secure the help he needed.

For years, I lived in fear whenever Robert was away, leaving me alone with our four young children, one of whom had cerebral palsy. Looking back now, I can understand that this fear was born from a complex mix of reasons, primarily the daunting challenges that came with caregiving. Nathan's condition placed tremendous physical and emotional demands on us, requiring constant attention and care. These responsibilities often made me doubt my own abilities, especially when I lacked the support of others.

Safety was a never-ending concern. Nathan's athetoid cerebral palsy meant unpredictable and involuntary movements, which kept me on high alert, ensuring he was never left unattended. Still, the underlying fear that he might accidentally hurt himself when I was alone with him gnawed at my peace of mind, leaving me uncertain about how to handle such situations.

Communication barriers only added to my anxiety. Nathan was nonverbal and couldn't express his needs or emotions, which created frustration for both of us. This challenge became even more pronounced when we were alone together, intensifying the feeling of helplessness.

The emotional toll of caregiving was relentless. Raising a child with a disability brought forth a whirlwind of complex emotions, including guilt, sadness, and a pervasive sense of isolation. This isolation became even more acute when I found myself alone with him, as it limited my opportunities to take breaks or seek emotional support from others.

Before long, I began experiencing caregiver burnout. At that time, it felt like I had nowhere to turn for support, understanding, or resources. There were no local support groups or educational materials to help me build my confidence and caregiving skills. This difficult experience ultimately shaped my advocacy work, as it underscored the importance of maintaining open communication and relying on a strong support network as crucial tools in managing my anxiety and providing the best possible care for my child. For a period, I experienced four of the five stages of the grieving process: denial, anger, bargaining, and depression[16]. However, it's important to note that this journey through grief was far from linear. Some days brought signs of progress, while others inundated me with intense emotions.

Upon later reflection, I realized that there was even more to it. Surrendering would have meant releasing hope, as if I were doubting God's capability to intervene and assist my child. Moreover, it would have unraveled everything I had believed about the pregnancy, making it feel like all our pain and struggles had been in vain. My faith couldn't withstand that blow, so I continued pressing forward.

I am not sure when the shift in my perspective began. I didn't notice at first that my focus gradually moved away from solely dwelling on the disability itself. Instead, it started to center on my faith. My prayers also changed; they became less about fixing Nathan and more about helping me see my child as God sees him.

Somewhere amidst all of this, the belief that God had a purpose for our lives began to reemerge. In my contemplation, I reflected on the fact that God had orchestrated Nathan's birth, determining his parents, family, and even the country of his birth. Given this, it seemed reasonable to conclude that there was a divine plan even in the midst of this disability.

With this revelation, a set of expectations surfaced—fueled by a strong belief that my son deserved support and abundant opportunities to develop and thrive like any other child. It became clear to me that he deserved happiness, a sense of belonging, to be a child and enjoy his childhood, and the chance to live his life to the fullest. This was the genesis of my mission to push back

---

16 Elisabeth Kübler-Ross, On Death and Dying (Scribner, 1969).

against established systems that said otherwise and challenge the prevailing stereotypes that created barriers to his inalienable right to attend school and learn with his typically developing peers.

This new commitment to inclusion and community involvement began when he was about two years old. Every decision we made regarding our interactions within the community was deliberate. Nathan was always by our side. Even when our compact car was too small to accommodate our family of six and his foldable wheelchair, we made multiple trips to accommodate his inclusion.

Whenever someone approached me for a chat, and Nathan was nearby, I would warmly say, "Nathan, say hi to so-and-so." Nathan would respond with a radiant smile, and it didn't take long before people started greeting Nathan before me. Some would even playfully comment that they had come over primarily to say hi to Nathan.

When his siblings received a birthday party invitation, it became understood that he would show up too. During their elementary school years, we had birthday celebrations at school for each child. Nathan would enthusiastically join their class festivities, and when it was his birthday, they would come to his class. Before long, children from his siblings' classes, who had gotten to know him, eagerly came to celebrate with him. These efforts initially brought me to the attention of others because soon, I began receiving invitations to speak at churches, including our own, as well as at early childhood schools and parent-teacher association meetings.

THE IMPORTANCE OF COMMUNITY
AND SUPPORT

During this particular phase of our journey, a significant lesson came to light—the paramount importance of community and support. This lesson was acquired through a rather arduous process: contending with prevailing societal norms that discouraged discussions about disabilities, the underdeveloped state of laws and services for children with disabilities, and the unfortunate practice of some professionals failing to educate parents about their child's disability in a manner that equips them to offer meaningful support within their home environment. Even as I conscientiously worked to integrate Nathan into our lives and deal with the stages of grief without professional support, I had a pervasive sense of isolation, even when I was in the company of others.

The sense of isolation was particularly pronounced within the confines of our church community. As a result, we made the decision to move to a smaller, more intimate congregation. We selected the church associated with the kindergarten and elementary school our children were enrolled in. Our choice was influenced by a previous experience that we had attended as first-time visitors, during which Nathan received personal recognition by name.

However, our initial hope was soon shattered. The Sunday school classes remained inaccessible, and despite our three-year tenure at the church during which both Robert and I actively served the community—my involvement included teaching Sunday school and vocational Bible school—no provisions were made for Nathan. His spiritual needs were consistently overlooked despite my repeated requests. I vividly recall a specific incident when I was fundraising to secure funds for Nathan's therapy sessions in the USA. I approached the church leadership for assistance, and while they offered verbal support and prayers, no tangible support or assistance was provided, ultimately causing the fundraiser to fall through. We ended up spending out of pocket for the fundraiser, which did not recover its cost.

But while I wasn't getting understanding and inclusion from my church community, individual members from other congregations extended their support. I'm immensely grateful to my friend and former coworker, Wendean, as well as her daughter, Lisa, who offered their shoulders to lean on during my most trying moments when I found it difficult to pray. I distinctly remember a particularly challenging period when we were struggling with depleted funds and limited food in the house. In an act of tremendous kindness, Wendean's son arrived at our doorstep bearing bags filled with groceries. She had been considerate in her selections, ensuring the children had milk, juices, and snacks. Additionally, she took the initiative to cook chicken and other meats, noting that she understood my busy schedule and hoped this gesture would be of assistance. It provided more help and comfort than I could adequately express at the time. It exemplified the practical embodiment of the concept of being "God's hands and feet on earth." It served as a powerful reminder that someone was thinking of us and our needs and that there were individuals who genuinely cared.

During this same period of adjusting to Nathan's diagnosis, the financial strain of Nathan's specialist visits and tests, coupled with my own choice to leave my job, made it impossible for us to continue paying our older children's school fees. It was a time of uncertainty and despair. My faith wavered, and I struggled to regain my footing.

Lisa, a certified elementary school teacher, was on a sabbatical from her teaching career when she learned about our predicament. However, upon hearing of our struggles, she selflessly offered her support to homeschool them until we could stabilize our situation. Even though our resources were meager, Lisa poured her heart and soul into teaching my children.

I'll never forget the countless moments of prayer we shared, where her support helped strengthen my faith. One of the most transformative experiences during this challenging time was our joint exploration of *The Purpose Driven Life* by Rick Warren. Through Lisa's guidance, I began to uncover qualities within myself that had remained hidden, such as being encouraging, empathetic, and compassionate. These revelations not only boosted my self-esteem but also enabled me to see the silver lining in even the most difficult circumstances. Lisa's selflessness not only provided my children with an education when we needed it most but also helped me rediscover my own worth. She became our guiding light in the midst of the storm, and for that, I will forever be grateful.

Wendean, Lisa, and their family have remained among my favorite people. During that period of our greatest need, they ministered to us, and the significant impact of that day continues to inspire my work to this day.

It took years for me to come to the realization that God doesn't promise us an easy life. What He promises is His presence with us, offering help and strength as we navigate the path we are called to walk. In our particular case, I can now see how He used our experiences to challenge stereotypes and inspire people to view Nathan (as well as others with disabilities) as unique creations of God, each possessing their own strengths and purpose.

One testimony that assured me of this came several years ago from a former coworker whom I knew from my pre-motherhood life. He is an economic analyst who, after getting reacquainted with me, Nathan, and my work, openly admitted that individuals with disabilities were essentially invisible to him until he became acquainted with our family. Observing how we interacted with Nathan served as a practical eye-opener for him, making him more aware of the presence of others with disabilities in the community. Some of these individuals, he realized, had gone unnoticed for years without a second thought. Interestingly, he was actively engaged in various national development projects and consistently integrated a disability perspective to ensure that policies and programs were inclusive of the needs of individuals with disabilities. In response, I believe that if my life and the challenges we've faced can positively impact even one person, then it has been entirely worthwhile.

TAKEAWAY

Understanding the concept of community within my faith took time. Initially, I expected support from my immediate church circle, and it was disheartening when it didn't materialize as I hoped. However, as time passed and individuals like Wendean and Lisa stepped in, a deeper lesson emerged: As believers in Christ, we all belong to the Christian community, and God chooses to use whom He chooses to use according to His divine plan. Therefore, it's not for me to dictate the source of my help; my role is to present my needs to God, and He will provide. It was a message of faith.

This experience amplified the teachings of Christ, emphasizing our role as vessels of His love in the world. It underscored that the brilliance of His love shines most brightly when we, as a united Christian community, join hands to serve others. This collective effort sends a compelling message that God's care extends to all, regardless of their abilities or disabilities.

Additionally, it underscores the point that the church plays a crucial role within the community to help address human needs and promote holistic healing. It's often more accessible for individuals to connect with a church within their own community, and most churches do a great job in this regard. However, when it comes to individuals with disabilities and their families, there is a notable gap in many churches—a lack of knowledge on how to work with these individuals practically. My prayer is that highlighting this gap in this book may open up a conversation for change in church communities.

CHAPTER 14

ACCEPTANCE'S LONG AND WINDING ROAD

The Evolution of Understanding

The day Nathan silently developed pneumonia and came perilously close to losing his life (once again) marked a significant turning point for me. It prompted my decision to resign from my job so that I could be at home with him. Up until that moment, we had hired a nurse to care for him while I went back to work, covering her expenses from our own pockets. At that time, I still viewed Nathan primarily through the lens of his diagnosis, believing that with a capable healthcare professional, we were leaving him in capable hands.

However, just a few months after my return to work, I picked back up my hectic travel schedule, often traveling to organize out-of-town corporate events. This was deeply stressful, as it meant being away from home for extended periods, often lasting up to a week at a time.

During the incident in question, I had been away for several days, and every time I called home, I found that Nathan was asleep, regardless of the time of day. The nurse caring for him had mentioned that he had a slight cold, and despite a persistent feeling that something more serious might be happening, I didn't push further.

However, in the midst of my trip, I decided to return home to check on Nathan personally. When I arrived, I noticed that he seemed groggy, his skin was flushed, and he had a low-grade fever. My schedule had me returning to Montego Bay the next morning, but a strong instinct compelled me to take him to see his pediatrician before I left as a precautionary measure. Little did I know that this would prove to be lifesaving. The doctor's examination confirmed my worst fears—he had developed a severe case of pneumonia. The X-ray provided a stark depiction of the situation, revealing that his left lung was perilously close to collapsing. Fortunately, we detected this just in the nick of time. The urgency of the situation was unmistakable, demanding immediate hospitalization.

We rushed him to the University Hospital of the West Indies (UHWI), but our experience was far from smooth. The initial intake process was frustratingly slow, requiring me to speak up multiple times before any urgency was given to begin his treatment. Throughout his week-long hospitalization, we encountered numerous challenges that added to the already difficult situation.

One significant challenge we encountered was the placement of my child in a children's ward that lacked bed rail guards, putting him at risk of falling off the bed. Additionally, the hospital staff responsible for preparing meals for him faced difficulties understanding his dietary needs. This led to instances where they sent food he couldn't swallow or even forgot to provide him with meals.

So, for the second time in his young life, we established a round-the-clock caregiving schedule to ensure there was always someone there to advocate for his needs. Nathan was just eighteen months old at this point, and with so much of his childhood still ahead of him, the immense challenges that lay ahead couldn't be ignored. It was clear that his health remained unpredictable, with the potential for critical situations that demanded my constant presence and attention as his primary caregiver.

However, despite the gravity of the situation, I found myself in a state of inner turmoil, wrestling with the idea of stepping away from my career. This decision represented a significant life shift with profound consequences for my personal and professional identity.

My career was more than just a means of earning a living; it was a defining element of my identity. Now, at this difficult crossroads, I faced conflicting pulls. On one hand, there was the allure of my career—a source of fulfillment, financial stability, and a sense of achievement. On the other hand, there was my child—a precious soul who needed me, with his well-being and development at the forefront of my heart.

Still, making the decision was easy; however, walking away on the last day proved to be the most challenging. As we celebrated at the send-off party, I couldn't help but notice all that I was leaving behind. I believed I would never again contribute to the world in the same capacity. Thoughts of the income we were losing (my income accounted for two-thirds of our household budget) weighed heavily on me, and the prospect of managing without it was undeniably frightening.

However, my initial reactions and perceptions about my child's condition had shifted. I had gained more knowledge and experience to understand his different disposition. The thought of what could have happened had I not come home tipped the scales and helped me to realize that I was being called to serve my son and family in a new capacity.

CHALLENGES AND MILESTONES

As I closed that chapter of my life on the last day of work, I wrestled with intense feelings of loss and uncertainty. It felt like I was bidding farewell to something essential I might never encounter again. Standing before the cake during the farewell celebration, I noticed a verse was inscribed on it: "You will go out in joy and be led forth in peace; the mountains and hills will burst into song before you, and all the trees of the field will clap their hands." Although I didn't fully grasp the significance of those words at the time, they evoked a blend of emotions—hope, encouragement, and a gentle reminder that unforeseen blessings and joys could accompany this new journey. The verse alluded to a promising path ahead, which was encouraging.

But, after leaving corporate Jamaica, I oscillated between acute moments of self-doubt, when I questioned the wisdom of my decision, and instances of deep conviction, when I felt I had made the right choice. It didn't make things any easier that some individuals who were not experiencing my reality felt compelled to offer their opinions, often stating that I had made a mistake. Their reasoning was that, with a child with a disability, I needed more financial resources, not less.

Some close to me perceived my new role as simply "becoming a housewife with plenty of spare time," while others viewed it as an irresponsible and foolish choice. The judgment and unsolicited advice from others added another layer of complexity to my journey of self-discovery and redefinition.

Indeed, while their judgments held some validity, this new path ushered in some of our most profound blessings. It allowed me to form a deeper connection with Nathan and his siblings in ways that would have remained elusive had I continued my employment. I had the opportunity to work with Nathan one-on-one, deepening my understanding of his disability and how I could support his development in the everyday moments of life. This time also allowed me to engage in research, which enriched my knowledge and spurred my personal growth. I learned to place greater trust and dependence on God. I unearthed reservoirs of creativity, faith, strength, resilience, courage, and boldness within myself that I had never known existed.

As I came to discover, acceptance was not a static destination but an ongoing journey filled with twists and turns. It required me to confront my fears and priorities, placing my child's well-being above all else. It was a path I had willingly chosen, acknowledging that it wouldn't be easy, but it ultimately led me to a profound understanding of love, sacrifice, and the resilience of the human spirit.

Another development of this time is that I became an avid pupil of my children. A pivotal moment occurred about a year after my resignation when I overheard my ten-year-old daughter, Adrianne, explaining to a complete stranger that Mommy was home because she got fired from her job. This moment made me keenly aware that the impact of my decision extended beyond just Robert and me; it also profoundly affected our children. It underscored the vital role of honest and age-appropriate communication, even for the family's youngest members. This realization prompted a shift in my approach, emphasizing the importance of keeping our children well-informed about significant life changes to nurture trust and understanding.

It also mentored the relationship with Dawn.

THE ROLE OF SUPPORT

Everyone should have a Dawn in their life! Dawn's friendship was a precious gift that began with a shared experience of exclusion. We met a year before my pregnancy with Nathan, and during a corporate event, I stood up for her when she faced unfair treatment. Our bond deepened when she learned about my pregnancy complications and called me every day, brightening my spirits with her warmth, care, and infectious laughter. When Nathan was born, Dawn came to visit me at the hospital despite her physical challenges. She brought infectious energy and good spirits to my bedside at the hospital, remaining a steadfast pillar of love and support while others faded away.

During the darkest days after Nathan's diagnosis, Dawn's understanding, drawn from caring for her older nephew with autism, allowed her to empathize deeply with the immense shock and burden I carried. She gave me space and time without taking offense when I withdrew from the world and her. Despite my initial resistance to her calls, Dawn stayed persistent, reaching out every day and leaving messages of love and hope. Over time, her persistence dissolved my barriers, and I became truly grateful that she never gave up on me.

Dawn's was the only shoulder I could lean on, where I knew I could freely express my fears and emotions, and she would genuinely listen and understand. Talking to her felt cleansing, as I knew she held everything I shared confidentially. Her wisdom surpassed her years, offering practical advice and insights that made my struggles feel more manageable. Our daily conversations became a light, something I eagerly looked forward to, and our bond deepened as we shared our life stories and sought strength through prayer and scriptures together.

Dawn imparted a profound perspective on viewing obstacles and challenges as "grace-growers"—opportunities for spiritual and personal growth and learning. Under her guidance, I came to know that Jesus cared deeply about every aspect of my life. Whether it was tending to Nathan's needs, playing with him and his siblings, preparing meals, doing laundry, or handling household chores, each responsibility I embraced as a mother and wife became an act of worship—an offering to God. This was deeply liberating.

Among the many conversations we shared, one stood out in particular. I confided in her about feeling like I was letting God down because I could no longer serve in the church due to my increased responsibilities with Nathan. She listened closely, and when I finished, she posed a thought-provoking question. She asked me if Nathan could bring me a glass of water if I were thirsty or rub my feet if they hurt. I responded with a gentle no. Then, she asked if he could call for help if I needed assistance, and again, I replied, "No."

With a warm smile, she asked me why I loved him. I replied, "I love him because he's a part of me and a reflection of the love between his father and me. He trusts me completely, and I am determined to be the person he can always rely on. Above all, he is my son, a precious gift in my life who has filled my heart with love beyond measure. I am grateful every day for the privilege of being his mother." Dawn chuckled, clapped her hands, and said, "Precisely. God loves you because He is love, not because of what you can do for Him. So, even if you never did anything else for the rest of your life, His love for you would never diminish."

Her words resonated deeply with me, and that conversation etched itself into my heart over the years. It became a transformative reminder to keep my perspective on love clear—to love unconditionally without expecting anything in return. This lesson refreshed and deepened my love for God, my family, my loved ones, and myself. It instilled in me a profound understanding of the boundless love surrounding us and how we can share that love wholeheartedly with others.

After Dawn shared that insightful golden nugget, she effortlessly transitioned from her role as a teacher to that of a dear friend, infusing our conversation with her infectious humor and melodious laugh. By the end of the phone call, my anxieties of earlier were long forgotten.

Sadly, Dawn passed away suddenly when Nathan was just four years old. Her absence left an immense void in our lives, and I deeply mourned her loss. Her support and friendship during my acceptance journey were invaluable, and I will forever cherish her unwavering encouragement and understanding. Her memory holds a special place in my heart, serving as a potent reminder of the profound impact of genuine friendship, especially during the most trying times.

TAKEAWAY

I use the stories in this chapter, particularly Dawn's, to underscore the profound importance of support in our lives as we raised Nathan. Dawn played an immensely significant role in my journey toward accepting my son's diagnosis, embracing my new path in life, and recognizing myself as a worthy child of God. She offered invaluable spiritual guidance, served as a dedicated prayer partner, and helped me unearth my purpose—to bring a fresh perspective to the world, particularly in assisting children with disabilities and their families to thrive.

Although she is no longer with us physically, Dawn's legacy of compassion, kindness, patience, joy, love, and faithfulness continues to resonate. It remains a perpetual source of encouragement for me to strive to be the type of friend she exemplified—consistent and unwavering in her support.

CHAPTER 15

THE DAY I MET MY SON

From Fear to Connection

Despite my sincere efforts to uphold my commitment to accepting my life as it was, doubts and uncertainties would often sneak into my mind, especially after challenging nights or health setbacks. Sometimes, Nathan's care needs got so overwhelming that it clouded my perspective and tested my resolve.

One area where this inner conflict was most evident was in my evolving perception of Nathan. Despite having moved into the acceptance phase of the stages of grief (denial, anger, bargaining, depression, acceptance), I still wrestled with anger and frustration due to the daily attitudinal and environmental barriers we faced. In response, I became defensive and occasionally displayed passive-aggressive behavior toward anything I perceived as signs of exclusion, ignorance, or unfair treatment. My expectations of systems to accommodate him became somewhat unreasonable, and, for a period, I became more of an advocate than a mother.

This focus dominated my conversations. Any questions about Nathan's well-being quickly shifted toward what he wasn't doing, what he didn't have, and what the government wasn't doing. I wasn't aware of how this constant complaining affected those around me. But my friend Dawn was paying attention. She was the first person courageous enough to help me recognize this pattern.

During one of our conversations, she inquired about how Nathan was doing, and I responded in the context of what was lacking. She listened for a while and then gently interrupted and reframed her questions, "Chrissy, I am not asking about his disability; I am asking about *him*. How is Nathan, the child, doing today?" I found myself in a state of confusion, struggling to understand what she meant by this question. Until that moment, I had never contemplated the positive aspects of my son's development. In fact, I was challenged because I couldn't readily identify them. Dawn aided me by clarifying further, "What was he doing when you left him at home? Was he awake and playing? What is his favorite toy he loves playing with the most? What activities bring him joy when he's with you? With his dad? With his siblings? What are his favorite foods?" To my astonishment, I found myself unable to respond to any of her inquiries. I didn't have the answers. I realized I could talk endlessly about his disability, how it affected him, and his daily care routines and challenges. I could discuss my dreams, hopes, and desires for him. Yet, I didn't truly know him as a person.

It was a humbling moment. I came to the realization that I had become so accustomed to focusing on the "dis-" in his disability that I had neglected to see the "abilities" that were still very much present in my child. Somehow, I had inadvertently failed to see Nathan as a complete person, often reducing him to his needs and challenges. I had become so overwhelmed by what he lacked that I had failed to fully recognize the child right in front of me, with his unique personality, gifts, and untapped potential.

Upon reflection, it became clear how my interactions with various healthcare, rehabilitation, and medical professionals had unintentionally shaped this view of my son, which obscured his "personhood." Every appointment seemed fixated on what he couldn't do. Standardized evaluations, designed to measure "normal" child development, compared him to predetermined milestones impossible for a child with multiple disabilities to meet, emphasizing deficits. These assessments also had limited scope, concentrating on challenges rather than strengths. Nathan's complex mix of abilities and challenges often eluded the assessments, hindering our understanding of his capabilities.

Communication barriers were another major hurdle. It hindered his ability to tell us what he knew. Further, these assessments lacked individualization and didn't account for his unique needs and learning style. Thus, this sole focus on deficits perpetuated negative labels, obscuring Nathan's true potential and strengths.

I found myself admitting to Dawn that I couldn't answer her questions because I didn't know any of the answers. She chuckled softly and said, "My dear, have you met your son? It is said that the eyes are the windows to one's soul. Go home today and look into Mr. Nathan's eyes. Go meet your son!"

I followed Dawn's advice and decided to act. When I returned home that day, I went straight to Nathan. He was seated in his stroller, watching TV. I greeted him and expressed my desire to talk. I turned off the TV, pulled up a chair, and swiveled his stroller to face me, making sure we were at eye level. Normally, interrupting him during his showtime would provoke a fuss, but surprisingly, he didn't react negatively. It felt like he understood the moment's importance.

"Nathan, I have something special in mind for us. Let's look into each other's eyes and see what we can discover together." As our gazes locked, time seemed to stand still. Usually, he struggled to maintain prolonged eye contact or focus on anything for more than a few seconds. But that day was different; his gaze held mine. I can't explain how, why, or how long we stayed that way, but his spirit suddenly shone through. It was as though everything else simply dissolved into the background, and in that moment, I saw him for the remarkable human being he truly was—beyond the confines of his physical appearance, a wondrous and fearfully made individual.

His eyes revealed a deep soul and spirit that transcended any physical limitations. I was captivated by the beauty of him—the way the whites of his eyes framed his brown irises, his long silky eyelashes, his perfectly arched eyebrows, and his beautiful olive complexion. As I stared into his eyes, I saw how they twinkled and danced with energy and joy, a subtle hint of mischief and curiosity. I noticed how he smiled with his eyes. It was an unforgettable moment of connection.

Everything that had defined him up to that point—CDH, hospitalization, and the CP diagnosis—seemed to melt away. My heart overflowed with love, joy, and gratitude as I gazed at him and exclaimed, "Hi, honey, I am your mother, and you are my wonderful, perfect son!" We both burst into laughter together, and as he gazed at me, his laughter and smile seemed to convey, "I know, Mom. I know."

Whenever I recount this story, I often reflect on how it marked the first time I met my son. Back then, Nathan was two and a half years old, and I deeply regretted my approach to him up to that point, which had been primarily clinical. All of his toys were functional, whether they were educational, therapeutic, or sensory. Every decision up to that moment was driven by the desire to fix him. I realized that I had missed experiencing the essence of the child. I had never celebrated either of his two birthdays. When I looked at him, all I could see were his limitations.

But that day changed everything. It transformed my perspective, reminding me that my child was a child first. From that point onward, in everything I did, I resolved to acknowledge, respect, and prioritize the child within him.

BREAKING BARRIERS

After meeting my son, it became challenging to return to the therapy service he was receiving, the school program he was involved in, and the neurologist we were seeing. It reset my goal of finding programs and professionals with a people-first approach to their work.

I found *Disability Is Natural* by Dr. Kathie Snow to be an essential resource during this transitional period. It helped me understand the power of our words in shaping attitudes and perceptions, molding the fabric of social policies, and influencing our day-to-day interactions with people. This book introduced me to the notion of people-first language, highlighting the importance of prioritizing the person over the disability.

As I embraced this fresh approach to seeing and talking about my son and his disability, it became strikingly evident how it systematically eliminated prejudiced and hurtful descriptions, guiding me toward a communication style that was more inclusive and deeply respectful when talking about and interacting with my child. However, what truly stood out was the remarkable impact of this approach on Nathan. Through the filter of our steadfast respect and complete acceptance, Nathan started to radiate greater confidence and belief in his intrinsic worth that transcended any limitations imposed by his disability.

The result of all this was that Nathan started seeing himself differently. His self-esteem soared, he experienced enhanced mental well-being, and refined his social skills. It was joyful to see Nathan grow into a more confident, resilient person. As a parent, this was all I ever wished for each of my children.

As I grew to know my son on a deeper level, I discovered that he was a truly remarkable and beautiful soul with a wealth of thoughts, feelings, and preferences. I marveled at his wit, and his disarming smile had the power to warm even the coldest heart. Nathan's sociability was evident as he eagerly interacted with new people, and his intuition seemed almost like a sixth sense— he could discern the genuine from the insincere. He knew when someone could benefit from his million-dollar smile.

As I observed him closely, I began to see how intelligent he was. He possessed a unique ability to teach himself things, finding innovative methods to communicate his needs in an entirely personal way. His will, determination, and indomitable spirit left me in awe. Nathan became one of my greatest teachers, showing me the importance of resilience, self-expression, and celebrating individuality.

Through him, I learned to appreciate the beauty of every person's uniqueness and the value of genuine connections. His infectious spirit brought joy and laughter into our lives, brightening even the darkest days.

As my son, he became not just my responsibility but also my inspiration. He helped me discover the depths of my own strength and capacity for love. He illuminated the path of acceptance, teaching me that the true essence of caregiving lies in recognizing and celebrating the person within, beyond any labels or limitations.

A New Beginning

It is truly fascinating how, through my interactions and learning from Nathan, my entire family reaped the benefits. Learning to see Nathan beyond the surface not only deepened my understanding of people but also taught me to look beyond others' behaviors and attitudes. As I expanded my mindset and personal growth, these lessons naturally extended into our family dynamics.

I discovered the power of listening more actively to each family member, cherishing the unique qualities and perspectives they brought to our lives. I learned to love more deeply, not just in words but through actions that reflected genuine care and support. Engaging more meaningfully with my children and loved ones became a priority as I understood the significance of fostering strong connections and nurturing meaningful relationships.

Together, we found joy in our family's "new normal." Embracing acceptance brought a sense of peace and contentment, allowing us to focus on the present and create beautiful memories in the process. Each moment became a treasure, and we celebrated the small victories and shared laughter even amidst challenges.

Nathan's influence went beyond the walls of our home, shaping how I approached my work with children and families. His journey taught me valuable lessons in compassion, patience, and empathy.

TAKEAWAY

In retrospect, I can now see how my preoccupation with my child's disability led to feelings of fear, anxiety, and an uncertain outlook for the future. The weight of stereotypes and misconceptions only added to this overwhelming sense. It seemed as though every system and every person we encountered only emphasized his disability, leaving little room for anything else. However, it was through the wisdom of Dawn that I experienced a transformative moment when I finally met my son on a deeper level. It marked the first time I connected with his spirit, realizing that there was nothing broken about it. His spirit was whole, vibrant, and beautiful. This was what transported me to see my child's humanity beyond the disability, filling my heart with love and understanding. This transformation from fear to connection taught me the profound importance of seeing the person before the disability.

Another pivotal lesson that emerged from this experience was the beginning of breaking down barriers, with the most significant being attitudinal. It's truly astonishing how a seemingly simple practice, such as using people-first language, could profoundly impact people's attitudes and behaviors. Before this transformational moment, I had encountered numerous barriers within myself and how others perceived my child's disability. Stereotypes and misconceptions had created a cloud of prejudice that hindered understanding. However, as I began to adopt people-first language and prioritize seeing the person before the disability, I witnessed a remarkable shift in how those around us responded to Nathan. Others became more inclusive and empathetic toward him. This lesson underscored the transformative power of language in breaking down attitudinal barriers and fostering a more compassionate and accepting society.

CHAPTER 16

A JOURNEY OF HOPE AND EMPOWERMENT

The Shift in Perspective

After the pivotal moments that shifted my perspective, as described in the previous chapter, I found myself in a better place of acceptance. It became clear that we couldn't return to the specialists we had been working with before because our views on disability were fundamentally misaligned. Their approach was medical, focusing on fixing the disability itself.

At the same time, mine had evolved into a social perspective, seeing the disability not as something inherent to my son but as a product of his environment. I was determined not to allow him to remain connected with professionals who lacked belief in his abilities and failed to recognize his potential beyond cerebral palsy. Equally, I was unwilling to engage in yet another conversation that would dismiss the importance of holding optimistic expectations. My goal was to surround him with healthcare providers and clinicians who exuded optimism and shared our vision for his future.

Ending the physical therapy (PT) sessions was an agonizing decision. I was acutely aware that the PT had taken us on as a special favor to the referring neurologist. Also, given that we couldn't find a local speech therapist (SLP) who specialized in working with kids like Nathan and the only pediatric occupational therapist (OT) had a daunting two-year waitlist, it felt fatalistic to give up the physical therapy service.

He was receiving PT services at home twice a week for an hour. However, the therapist's choice of a neurodevelopmental approach made the decision clear to us. This approach involved structured exercises and activities designed to stimulate specific neurological pathways and enhance motor skills.[17] While this approach was beneficial, it proved to be quite challenging for Nathan as it entailed rigorous exercise drills. He vehemently disliked these sessions and strongly resisted the therapist's efforts.

As I struggled with the decision to terminate the sessions, one day, in a moment of frustration, Nathan clenched his tiny fist around the therapist's hair and yanked out a handful. It was a stark and painful reminder that this therapy wasn't truly benefiting him (or her), and I realized I had been deceiving myself by thinking it was better than nothing. After discussing it with Robert, we summoned the courage to make the tough call and discontinue the treatment.

The following day, I settled down at my computer, armed with a pen and an empty sheet of paper, and prayed for guid-

17 Lydia Furman, "Neurodevelopmental Therapy (NDT)—What is it and Does It Work?" AAP Journal, May 24, 2022, **https://publications.aap.org/journal-blogs/blog/20461/Neurodevelop-mental-Therapy-NDT-What-is-it-and-Does.**

ance. Since I hadn't found anyone locally, I knew I needed to look overseas, but I wasn't sure where. Then, like a beacon of inspiration, the idea struck me to reach out to my youngest sister, who resided in Miami. I called her and asked if she knew anyone with a child with cerebral palsy, and to my surprise, she did. She quickly provided me with the contact information for the developmental pediatrician her friend took her son to, and without hesitation, I made an appointment. This marked the beginning of a phase I like to refer to as the "Ray of Hope," which I will share more about shortly.

Obtaining referral support proved to be a challenging endeavor. Nathan's pediatrician was supportive and accommodating upon learning of our decision, readily providing the necessary documentation. However, our experience with the physical therapist was quite the opposite. She exhibited hesitation and skepticism and even suggested that pursuing this path would waste money and time, with no promise of a different outcome. Nevertheless, I pressed ahead, unwavering in my determination to pursue this course of action despite the doubts and discouragement.

Financing the trip was another hurdle. However, Robert's parents got wind of our plans and generously contributed the funds required to help cover the costs. Two months after ending his services in Jamaica, Nathan, Adrianne, and I boarded a flight to Miami, all set to meet with this new developmental pediatrician.

THE SEARCH FOR ANSWERS

This doctor's appointment marked another significant turning point that reshaped my perspective once again. Right from the moment we entered the parking lot, I was struck by something truly extraordinary—accessibility was evident everywhere. As we sat in the waiting room, my eyes were drawn to these beautiful children in their tiny wheelchairs, cheerful colors, and even their AFOs[18] adorned with beloved cartoon characters. They radiated hope, happiness, and the unmistakable essence of childhood.

Then, I looked at Nathan, seated in an oversized baby stroller that offered him minimal support. He was dressed in somber, dark clothing, devoid of the light and colorful attire I had chosen for his siblings at his age. A sense of melancholy washed over me as I wondered why Nathan and other children in Jamaica couldn't access this level of support and care.

Inside, the doctor's office immersed us in the practical aspects of a people-first approach. The doctor chose to sit with us on a vibrant playmat tucked away in one corner of her office, positioning herself at eye level with Nathan. Every time she addressed me, she would turn to him and say, "So, Nathan, I'm explaining this to Mommy. It's to help you do this and that." Nathan would respond with an infectious smile as if he understood every word.

As the appointment neared its end, she handed me a stack of referrals for evaluations for occupational, speech, and physical therapy, ophthalmology, audiology, nutrition, and orthotics. I was taken aback because, aside from her, I had no knowledge of any other specialists or even where to begin seeking appointments. Time was also against us; we had just three weeks.

I returned to the car to discuss the outcome of the appointment with my mother, who had accompanied us. In her customary style, she invited me to pray with her on the matter. When we were done, I went back inside, as the doctor's office was situated in the pediatric wing of a rehabilitation hospital. I wanted to see

---

18 The term "AFOs" stands for ankle-foot orthoses.

which of the services were available and whether they were able to accommodate him.

That was the moment when the first in a series of miracles began to unfold. I was conversing with the physical therapist, discussing how her earliest appointment was six months away, when the phone suddenly rang. She excused herself to answer it and returned with a beaming smile, sharing the unexpected, good news. The caller had been her 11:30 a.m. client, who had just canceled their appointment. If we were available, she could see us now.

Before I could fully process this stroke of luck, the occupational therapist, who happened to be nearby, approached us. She conveyed that the same client who had canceled with the physical therapist had also canceled their appointment with her. This meant she could see Nathan immediately after our session with the physical therapist. It was a remarkable turn of events, teaching me the importance of the scripture, "Ask and it will be given to you; seek and you will find; knock and the door will be opened to you. For everyone who asks receives; the one who seeks finds; and to the one who knocks, the door will be opened."[19]

That day and week, it was like the universe itself was on our side, conspiring to give us that ray of hope. Once they heard our story, both therapists went out of their way to call their colleagues and get us scheduled for evaluations. People even reached out to us after their workday was over or during their lunch breaks. Somehow, the PT and OT found time to see Nathan for half an hour thrice weekly. They also took the time to teach me how to help him with certain skills.

19 Matthew 7:7–8 (NIV)

It didn't stop there. The orthotist found time to see him, measuring him for AFOs and a body vest to help stabilize and support him. He was leaving on vacation before we departed for Jamaica, but somehow, he expedited the production of the braces and even arranged to meet with us on his way to the airport for the fitting. Since we had no insurance and were paying out of pocket, the PT gave us a tip to tell the billing department that we were "out of pocket," which got us a discount on the services. This strategic decision proved to be a game changer, enabling us to allocate our funds wisely. We were able to not only cover the costs of PT and OT treatment sessions but also invest in essential therapeutic aids. Additionally, it afforded us the opportunity to purchase new clothing for Nathan and acquire some delightful toys that were purely for fun, enriching his life and making it even more enjoyable.

One of the most remarkable discoveries was the use of a play-based approach. I remember feeling a bit anxious as I watched the physical therapist secure Nathan into a small gait trainer.[20] At first, he seemed resistant, but everything changed when she placed a ball in front of him and encouraged him to kick it. To my amazement, he eagerly kicked the ball, and for the entire session, he had an absolute blast while simultaneously engaging in weight-bearing and mobility exercises.

I was impressed with how the different therapists seamlessly incorporated play into their therapy sessions, making them effective and genuinely enjoyable for Nathan. Over the few weeks we spent there, I marveled at the rapid development of Nathan's physical skills and his achievement of several important milestones. The therapists' creative techniques and adaptable

---

20 A mobility device designed to assist individuals with impaired mobility.

approach fostered a nurturing environment that allowed him to thrive. They also provided his first home management plan for us to implement when we returned home. It was a moment of empowerment and newfound confidence in my ability to support my child.

The experience of working with multidisciplinary clinicians opened my eyes to what clinical practices should ideally involve and what families should expect from these services. It became clear that certain fundamental aspects, such as receiving a written evaluation report and a comprehensive treatment plan, were standard procedures in the US but were notably absent in our experiences with physical therapy in Jamaica. I felt a deep sense of responsibility to empower and inform other parents about these crucial rights and expectations in the world of healthcare and therapy.

Our journey to Miami, initially taken on faith, ultimately became the spark for a brand-new chapter in our lives. I was resolute in my determination to share all the invaluable lessons I had learned and to become an advocate to enable Jamaica's laws and policies on the inclusion of people with disabilities. Such changes would help pave the way for adopting these best practices that increase the level of support for children with disabilities in our homeland. I firmly believe in the fundamental right of every child to have access to the care and support they require, not just to survive but to truly thrive.

THE BIRTH OF THE NATHAN EBANKS FOUNDATION

Upon returning home, I took decisive action to secure better support for Nathan. Recognizing the importance of collaboration,

I strengthened my partnership with Nathan's pediatrician, providing them with copies of the evaluation and treatment plans. I also went in search of a general education setting for him.

A few weeks later, an incredible opportunity presented itself when the principal of his sibling's preparatory school offered to enroll Nathan as a student. The only condition was that we had to find, train, and provide a special needs aide to accompany him to school. I jumped at the opportunity, seeing its potential to provide Nathan with a more normalized education.

The search for therapy services remained a formidable challenge. At that point, I had managed to locate several physical and speech therapists. However, every time I approached them, the response was disappointingly consistent: they claimed they couldn't accommodate Nathan's needs or promised to call me back but never did. This left me curious and concerned, prompting me to dig deeper into the issue.

Much to my dismay, I came to realize that I had acquired an unfortunate reputation within the close-knit community of clinicians. I was unfairly labeled as a "problem" parent solely because I had the audacity to ask probing questions and request information regarding their policies for providing written evaluation reports and treatment plans. This negative perception circulated, blocking Nathan from accessing any of these services. It was astonishing to think that access to services could be blocked for a vulnerable two-year-old child simply because I advocated for my child's essential needs.

But, as disheartening as these experiences were, they ultimately served a higher purpose. If I had effortlessly found all the services Nathan needed, our story would have taken a vastly different turn, and the Nathan Ebanks Foundation might never have come into existence. In retrospect, I realized that these trials and challenges had a profound significance. They weren't intended to harm us but to prepare us for a greater mission.

In 2007, the Nathan Ebanks Foundation was born out of a sense of concern, responsibility, duty, and a profound desire to give back. My vision was clear—a future where no family would experience the isolation and helplessness we once experienced. Instead, they would discover a nurturing community, essential resources at their fingertips, and a powerful voice to advocate for their rights and needs.

TAKEAWAY

I only came to understand the gifts that these experiences released in hindsight. During the trials themselves, I was always angry, overwhelmed by pain, and filled with disbelief. It was nearly unbearable to witness professionals treating my son in a manner that appeared to hinder his potential rather than nurture it.

But as time passed, a different perspective began to emerge. It became increasingly clear that the events guiding us along this path couldn't be coincident. It felt as though a higher power, the hand of God, was at work, intricately orchestrating the circumstances of our lives. It seemed that I was being shaped and molded to accumulate knowledge, insights, and experiences and utilize them for a greater purpose.

Because of this phase of our journey, I found my true calling: to offer support and resources that leave a lasting, meaningful impact on the lives of others walking a similar path. As I reflect on it all, I now recognize the compassionate understanding, empathy, creativity, resilience, and determination that these experiences unlocked within us—a hidden gift in disguise.

CHAPTER 17

AWAKENING TO PURPOSE

Taking Action and Living with Purpose

Nathan's initial experience in the first level of kindergarten was truly wonderful. The early childhood teacher, may her memory be a blessing, possessed genuine compassion and a calling to work with this particular population. Her heightened sensitivity and awareness were influenced by having a nephew with disabilities. Every day I arrived to pick up Nathan from school, she would remark, "Mrs. Ebanks, it was a pleasure having Nathan today. I keep asking myself, where are these 'special needs' I keep hearing about? All I see in him is what is typical for his age." Her words alleviated my concerns about his disability and reassured me about the nurturing and inclusive environment she was creating.

However, at the end of the school year, he transitioned to another kindergarten level with a completely different teacher.

This new teacher appeared to be apprehensive about his disability and lacked the training and experience to relate to him effectively. Consequently, she made choices about his participation based on what she believed he couldn't do, thereby restricting his opportunities. This led to a growing disparity between him and his peers, causing the initial experimental arrangement to unravel. The teachers frequently sought my assistance during training sessions, as they were uncertain about how to provide him with effective support. Since there were no special education teachers at the school, and they were not trained in special education themselves, I willingly assumed this role.

He moved into a new class at the end of that school year. Unfortunately, before he even arrived, the new teacher had already decided that she couldn't teach him and didn't want him in her class. This marked the beginning of a tumultuous year.

Because his previous teacher never worked with him in any capacity, he entered the new class as a nonverbal student with no established method of communication. His struggles with maintaining focus for more than a few seconds had intensified, making it challenging for him to engage in seatwork, which was now required at this higher grade level.

Compounding the issue was the fact that he was the only child in the school with multiple disabilities. This lack of diversity in the student population led to a one-size-fits-all approach to teaching. He was taught and tested using standardized methods designed for his typically developing peers, a recipe for disastrous performance.

The school's rigid structure further exacerbated the situation. He became isolated from his peers and virtually invisible in the classroom. No one spoke to him, not even his classmates; they directed their questions and comments about him to his aide, right in his presence. The absence of friends to connect with left him profoundly unhappy.

The teacher's persistent complaints to the principal about not wanting him in her class led to a meeting. During this meeting, the principal made it explicit that his removal from the school would be considered unless I could offer the necessary training. I felt trapped and uncertain about how to proceed.

In my search for a local special education teacher trained to work with students with multiple disabilities, I came up empty-handed. Additionally, I wasn't even sure about the specific training required. In line with my established practice, I turned to prayer for guidance. Afterward, I began extensive online research, scouring the internet for specialists in North America who might be willing to come to Jamaica to provide the necessary training. My determination remained unwavering despite knowing that I lacked readily available funds to pay such a person.

During my research, I stumbled upon several special education speakers bureaus. These bureaus brought together a diverse range of speakers, including educators, researchers, administrators, parents of children with disabilities, and professionals in special education. I was elated to discover that they offered workshops and training sessions that provided invaluable insights, practical strategies, and evidence-based approaches for supporting students with multiple disabilities in the classroom.

Motivated by this discovery, I promptly contacted multiple speakers, sharing my situation's details and intentions. To my delight, I received swift and encouraging responses. Each person praised my courage and determination in seeking help for my son. However, despite their positive feedback, I was disheartened to learn that all the speakers were fully booked for the year.

Fortunately, one professor kindly referred me to a colleague through a connecting email. A chain of referrals continued, and it was through the sixth person that I finally met Senta Greene, whose work and passion focused on the inclusion of children with multiple disabilities in educational and community settings.

Connecting Across Borders to Build Bridges of Support

The conversations I had with various individuals before connecting with Senta played a pivotal role in shaping my understanding of what I aimed to achieve—meaningful inclusion of Nathan in his general education classroom. The initial telephone conversation with Senta stretched over several hours. She listened attentively as I poured out my story, frustrations, and hopes during that time. She asked questions along the way, seeking clarity and extracting the information needed to understand the depth of my objectives.

When she finally began speaking, I was left utterly stunned. It was as though she had grasped the very essence of our situation and precisely what was needed. She proceeded to share several anecdotes of her own experiences that offered potential solutions to what I was seeking. The connection between us felt seamless as if she intimately knew Jamaica and me on a deeper level beyond our initial meeting. Tears welled in my eyes throughout that first meeting and several subsequent ones. She shared a philosophy that perfectly matched what I had been seeking in the professionals I wanted to collaborate with: a dedication to a people-first approach, the practice of people-first language, and a personal commitment to child-centered planning[21].

Senta's mentorship began on the first day. She discussed that inclusion is a philosophy that promotes equality, diversity, and the full participation of children with disabilities in all aspects of society. It recognizes that every child has the right to live a fulfilling life and reach their full potential, regardless of their abilities or differences.

It felt as if we had known each other for years, transcending borders to build bridges of support. Her organization's motto, "To touch the heart of a child is to touch the soul of a nation," truly came alive in our partnership. She stood by my side, offering compassion, empathy, and professional wisdom as we designed and implemented our first inclusive education workshop, "Teaching Students with Disabilities in Mainstream Classrooms." This comprehensive two-day workshop included a hands-on component, during which Nathan and other children with disabilities actively engaged, demonstrating the practical strategies we were imparting.

Nathan thrived on the attention, and his charm endeared him to the workshop attendees. This event marked a groundbreaking milestone as the first of its kind in Jamaica and was a resounding success. Subsequently, we collaboratively organized seven annual inclusive education conferences, conducted numerous customized training sessions for various schools and educational institutions, hosted community events, and provided consulta-

---

21 Child-centered planning is an educational and support approach that revolves around tailoring individualized learning or support plans for children by placing the child at the core of decision-making. It prioritizes the unique needs, strengths, and goals of each child, encourages inclusion in mainstream settings, fosters collaboration among educators and professionals, sets specific and measurable goals, involves ongoing assessment, and empowers children to have a voice in their own education and support planning, promoting a holistic approach to child development and education.

tions. Notably, we also established a Trainer of Trainers program for the Ministry of Education, modeled after the success of that initial workshop.

CHANGING A NATION BY TOUCHING THE HEART OF A CHILD

Throughout our partnership, I heavily relied on Senta's expertise over the years. She skillfully guided me in understanding the cultural context of our situation from multiple angles—personal, situational, environmental, global, and domestic. Through her guidance, I came to appreciate that there is a valuable role for both parents and parent-professionals[22] alike. This revelation helped me find my rightful place, a seat at the table as a parent-professional, with the role of improving the quality of services and support available to children with disabilities and their families. I discovered that my distinctive blend of personal insights and professional knowledge helped me foster more effective collaboration and mutual understanding within special education and disability advocacy.

Senta's mentorship, which gradually evolved into a deep and enduring friendship over the years, played a pivotal role in our collective achievements as a family and ignited a nationwide movement. She possessed a remarkable talent for unlocking the potential within individuals, enabling them to perceive things from fresh and innovative perspectives. I witnessed this transformative ability on numerous occasions during our years of collaboration. We would enter meetings with diverse stakeholders, and before long, those who had not been working together found

---

22 A parent-professional is someone who has personal experience as a parent or caregiver of a child with special needs or disabilities and also possesses professional expertise in disability, education, or related fields.

themselves engaged in meaningful and purposeful dialogues, resulting in groundbreaking collaborations.

One of my earliest memories that testified to my divine connection with Senta occurred on her first visit to Jamaica for our collaborative workshop. We had known each other for about six months when she, accompanied by her husband Russell, landed in Jamaica. Robert and I picked them up from the airport, and within minutes, she and I were laughing and finishing each other's sentences as if we were long-time friends. Russell turned to Robert and asked, "How long have these two ladies known each other?" To onlookers, including our husbands, our instant connection was so palpable that it seemed as if we had been friends for a lifetime.

During the same trip, my pastor led a spirited devotion to bless the day's proceedings. At one point, I looked over at Senta, realizing that I hadn't informed her about this aspect of how I did things. In fact, I hadn't discussed my Christian faith with her at all, as the topic had never come up. I noticed Senta stepping out several times during the devotion, but she always returned shortly afterward. I assumed she might have been uncomfortable with the blend of spiritual and professional elements. However, at the end of that day, as I drove her back to her hotel, she confided about how deeply the short service moved her. She explained that she was originally from the South and found the spirit of the session similar to what she was used to growing up. Each time she went outside, she called her mother back in California so that she could listen in on the prayers.

That was the moment when I realized that we were kindred spirits. The workshop had blessed her as deeply as it had blessed me and every other participant. Even though it was only the first day, accolades began pouring in from the attendees. The following day, we had a surge of new registrants, as those who had attended on day one shared the dynamic and transformative effects of the workshop. By the end of the three days, Senta and I had become close allies—not only as parents but also as individuals dedicated to making a meaningful difference in the lives of marginalized and excluded children.

Interestingly, with sponsorship from Robert's company covering some of the costs, including Senta's expenses, I extended a scholarship offer to Nathan's teacher and several others from his school, as I believed (at the time) that they were the primary reason for hosting the workshop. However, none of them attended, and I took it personally for a while, especially as, just a week after the workshop, I was once again summoned to a meeting and informed that the teacher couldn't effectively teach Nathan.

Years later, I came to realize that they had inadvertently sparked a movement that extended far beyond my initial intentions, benefiting thousands of children in Jamaica. Senta and I collaborated for a decade, and eventually, the school principal attended one of our workshops and affirmed its excellence. However, by that time, Nathan had moved on to another institution, and the impact of our work had already begun reshaping the conversation and thought processes regarding the effective inclusion of children with disabilities, even in resource-constrained settings.

TAKEAWAY

The way I met Senta and immediately felt a deep connection with her spoke of a spiritual bond. It was as though she had been perfectly prepared for the evolving mission in Jamaica, with her interests, training, and experiences aligning beautifully. After that first workshop, it felt like a major piece of the puzzle had fallen into place with remarkable synchronicity. While the path ahead was unclear, working with Senta refocused my eyes to see the hidden gifts, talents, and abilities I never knew existed within me.

The Scripture wisely reminds us, "As iron sharpens iron, so one person sharpens another,"[23] alluding to the inherent power of divine partnerships. These alliances harness the synergy, guidance, shared values, and resilience of individuals united by purpose. Rooted in a sense of higher purpose and trust, they inspire transformation, fostering personal growth and a lasting impact that extends beyond the individuals involved. Whether spiritual or symbolic, divine partnerships embody the potential for positive change and unity in the pursuit of shared goals.

---

23 Proverbs 27:17 (NIV)

CHAPTER 18

THE POWER OF UNCONDITIONAL ACCEPTANCE

The Healing Impact of Unconditional Acceptance

With no one to guide me and no existing literature to shed light on the path our journey raising Nathan would take, I held the belief that once I had embraced his disability and my role as a parent-professional assisting others, everything would proceed smoothly and seamlessly. But as I would soon discover, life rarely adheres to such simplicity. Accepting this new normal and integrating it into our daily lives were two distinct challenges. I quickly recognized the intricacies and encountered unexpected twists and turns. I learned that there were hidden layers that challenged my acceptance and drew out a deeper level of commitment.

Whether it was the struggle of lifting Nathan and his wheelchair up the classroom steps (with no ramp installed after three years), the frequent summons to the principal's office for yet another reason why he couldn't continue at the school, or the stark realization that my personal income fell short of providing for my family as I would have liked, these circumstances had the capacity to unsettle me, edging me closer to the point of giving up.

To make matters worse, I had been running the Nathan Ebanks Foundation entirely on my own for three years since its inception. My daily interactions with parents, who were often at their breaking point, left me emotionally drained. It was like peeling back the bandage from an open wound—simultaneously painful and healing. There were days when I couldn't hold back tears as they shared their stories of hardship. And the fact that I was still dealing with many of the same struggles made it all the more challenging. So, every week, I carried my worries with me to church. I ended up earning the title of "Mom is always crying in church" from my daughter Adrianne because I felt utterly powerless in my desire to provide the extensive help I longed to offer.

My speaking ministry was also rapidly expanding, sometimes faster than I could manage. Yet, there were moments during these engagements when my emotions ran deep, and the tears would flow, making it increasingly challenging to continue speaking.

I vividly recall a particular instance during which a popular radio talk show host posed a question that left me utterly speechless. He asked why the government (of Jamaica) should allocate resources to educate children with disabilities who, in his view, couldn't contribute to society, especially when there were "perfectly normal children who needed help." I stumbled through my response on live air, shocked by his statement. It compelled me to dig deeper to understand children's rights, human rights, and the obligations of governments in ensuring the success of all children. This knowledge was my armor for the next encounter. As expected, this question continued to surface in subsequent interviews. It became a powerful tool to emphasize our message that inclusion was not a privilege but the right of every child.

Juggling this kind of high-demand and unpaid work without a dedicated staff, any formal training in disability matters, or adequate funding amid a passive-aggressive environment, all while fulfilling my responsibilities to my son and family, was often an overwhelming challenge.

One crushing incident occurred when I was hosting our annual special education workshop. My friend Wendean came on as a volunteer to help with sponsorship fundraising. Her feedback was disheartening as she recounted the negative responses from some of the companies I had approached. The director of one company specializing in the sale of medical and therapeutic equipment took issue with my message. She complained to Wendean that she would not support my organization because I gave parents false hope by suggesting therapy support or adaptive equipment could improve their children's lives. According to this individual, who worked in healthcare and owned the company, my role should be encouraging parents to accept their children's disabilities as an inevitable fate.

I also couldn't help but notice how sharing some of the everyday challenges faced by children with disabilities made some audiences uncomfortable whenever I spoke. I have to admit that this initial discomfort bothered me. However, I soon came to realize that for genuine and meaningful change to take place, we all needed to push past our comfort zones and confront the uncomfortable truths. Progress simply couldn't happen unless we were willing to acknowledge the real issues at hand and truly understand what was required to address them.

The weight of being the sole parent voice in this endeavor was undeniably heavy. However, naming the foundation after my son, Nathan Ebanks, was a deliberate choice. Whenever I felt like giving up, I would think of him; that thought alone was enough to keep me going. I could never give up on him, and that commitment served as a constant source of motivation.

One evening, I found myself in a vulnerable conversation with a close friend. She praised my commitment and efforts in peeling back the layers of issues facing children with disabilities in real and insightful ways. However, despite her words of encouragement, I struggled to see that what I did mattered. I doubted my own abilities, convinced that I lacked the academic credentials for the job. Moreover, in one of the national working groups I participated in as a parent-professional volunteer, a leading healthcare specialist consistently referred to me as "the housewife." This triggered deep-seated insecurities that had persisted since I left corporate Jamaica and amplified what is commonly known as the "impostor syndrome."[24]

I confided in my friend about these doubts and insecurities, describing how it seemed like I was dedicating my time, energy, and limited resources to a cause that I couldn't seem to make headway in. The burden of it weighed heavily on my conscience, and I couldn't shake the feeling that I was taking away from my family and placing undue pressure on my husband, Robert.

---

24 Impostor syndrome is a psychological phenomenon in which individuals, despite external evidence of their competence, skills, or achievements, have persistent feelings of inadequacy and a fear of being exposed as frauds or impostors. Impostor Syndrome can lead to self-doubt, anxiety, and a lack of self-confidence, which can impact both personal and professional aspects of a person's life.

She gently reminded me of the timeless wisdom found in Galatians 6:9–10 (NIV): "Let us not become weary in doing good, for at the proper time we will reap a harvest if we do not give up. Therefore, as we have opportunity, let us do good to all people, especially to those who belong to the family of believers." These verses became a mantra I often repeated whenever I felt discouraged.

For several months, I devotedly combed through the Bible for scriptures that resonated with my circumstances during my morning devotional time. I transcribed them onto cue cards and strategically placed them in various spots in my daily life: my computer screen, closet door, and bathroom mirror. These visual reminders became my unwavering companions, assuring that the wisdom encapsulated within these verses held a prominent place in my thoughts, guiding my decisions throughout the day. Every choice, every tear, and every problem I found solutions to contributed to my healing journey from the trauma.

ENHANCING RELATIONSHIPS THROUGH ACCEPTANCE

Nathan was about seven years old by this time. I had become known as a passionate advocate for children with disabilities and their families in Jamaica and was often called upon by the media to speak on various issues for this population. Nathan and Robert joined in, actively participating in the programs of the Nathan Ebanks Foundation. Nathan, in particular, shone like a brilliant star during these engagements. He loved these opportunities as they tapped into his social strengths, and the audience loved interacting with him. Naturally, we approached his involvement with great care, ensuring he had the right preparation and support for engaging with the audience.

I also discovered that fully embracing acceptance enhanced my relationship with myself. This enabled me to discuss my challenges and successes openly. Recognizing that, much like I was in the beginning, many individuals working in local nonprofit organizations serving children with disabilities lacked formal training, I sought and got a grant from an international training and support charitable organization from the United Kingdom to carry out capacity-building for these organizations. We established a basic provider certification training program that brought occupational, speech, and physical therapists to Jamaica to provide hands-on training to improve the care and management of the children.

At the end of the first phase of the training, the director of the leading local disability support nonprofit approached me. She candidly admitted that initial impressions had painted me as self-promoting. However, after observing my actions over the duration of the workshop and closely listening to my words, she realized that these judgments were unfounded. She said she could see that I was authentic and following God's leading. Though I wasn't aware that she had prejudged me, she apologized for it. Since then, we have partnered together on many initiatives, and our relationship has evolved into a sincere friendship.

I've come to understand that disability is an intrinsic part of our human experience, showcasing our shared humanity and the resilience that stems from our interconnectedness. I've also realized that God employs others to assist me, just as He employs me to support others, and that together, we constitute the solution. That's why, for me, relationships are such a crucial element of this work.

SELF-ACCEPTANCE AND PERSONAL GROWTH

Unconditional acceptance of our life circumstances was a crucial cornerstone in cultivating self-acceptance, ultimately playing a pivotal role in nurturing my personal and professional growth and development. The turning point on my journey of self-discovery arrived when I fully embraced vulnerability. That was when I cast off the suffocating cloak of shame that had burdened me for so long and began to see my challenges as integral to my journey. It became glaringly evident how I had distanced myself from my authentic self, consistently relegating my own needs and aspirations to the background, all under the misguided notion that it was my duty to do so.

One ordinary day, my wise-beyond-her-years daughter, Adrianne, posed a simple yet profound question: "Mommy, why have you stopped smiling?" Her innocent inquiry opened the door to deeper self-reflection. Pastor Rick Warren's book, *The Purpose Driven Life*,[25] became a vital resource that helped me reconnect with my true self and understand that I was shaped for a purpose, including parenting my son and carrying out my work. I studied the book with Wendean and Lisa and was pleasantly surprised to discover that everything I was doing aligned perfectly with my core values: faith, family, compassion, contribution, and honesty.

TAKEAWAY

It wasn't until several years down the road that I truly grasped the remarkable gifts that come with unconditional acceptance. I discovered deep healing value in talking and writing about these

---

25 Rick Warren, The Purpose-Driven Life: What on Earth Am I Here for? (Grand Rapids, Michigan: Zondervan, 2002).

traumatic experiences. Every time I opened up and told my story, I was on a path to healing. I gained fresh insights and realized that this process was a powerful way to emotionally process and make sense of my past. It allowed me to transform from a passive victim into an empowered overcomer. Putting my experiences into words brought relief from the emotional distress that had haunted me for so long. Moreover, it helped me develop coping strategies and enhanced my ability to manage my emotions.

Beyond the personal benefits, sharing my story also connected me with a supportive community of individuals who offered empathy and encouragement. Storytelling became an integral part of my journey, enabling me to integrate fragmented memories into a coherent narrative and regain control over my own story.

CHAPTER 19

JOURNEY COMPANIONS

Where Do We Find Journey Companions?

Having journey companions in the context of raising a child with disabilities means having individuals or a network of people who provide support, understanding, and companionship throughout our parenting journey. These remarkable companions are intimately involved in our experiences, sharing in the joys and struggles we encounter. They offer not just emotional support but practical assistance, too, helping us navigate the intricate landscape of healthcare, education, advocacy, and daily life. I've personally never felt this need for companionship more profoundly than after Nathan was born. As I would soon discover, companions can take many forms, including family members, friends, support groups, professionals, and educators, all of whom deeply empathize with our family's situation. They play an indispensable role in reducing feelings of isolation, offering valuable guidance, and joining in the celebration of milestones and successes. These journey companions provide a sense of unity and shared purpose, making the challenging journey of raising a child with disabilities more manageable and far less daunting.

As Nathan continued to grow, a new set of challenges emerged. It often felt like for every problem I managed to solve, two or three more would surface. This could be incredibly frustrating at times. What added to the complexity was that I was still figuring out what inclusion could truly look like in Jamaica, especially given the absence of many specialists and clinicians who were needed to support this process. I found myself creating a model of inclusion for Nathan that simply didn't exist anywhere, and as I watched his early childhood years slip away, I couldn't help but feel a growing sense of anxiety.

During this phase, Senta remained one of the pillars of strength in my life. However, there were other areas that now required attention, particularly in the realm of speech therapy services. This wasn't just for Nathan but also for many of the children whose parents turned to the Nathan Ebanks Foundation for guidance and support.

So, I prayerfully undertook another search. This is when I met Dr. Fay E. Brown. My high school friend Karaine in Connecticut noticed I was becoming frustrated again. Although I didn't personally know Karaine during our high school years, we graduated in the same class. She served as the president of our social media alumni group and later became a close friend when we reconnected more than two decades later. She had been a steadfast supporter, and recognizing that I was in a vulnerable state, she kindly arranged for me to visit her, stepping away from everything and taking time to clear my head.

During the visit, one of the days I was there, she arranged for me to join her in a cold call to Dr. Brown. Dr. Brown generously gave us a few minutes of his time before he had to head to a meeting. However, being an educational psychologist born in Jamaica, she was deeply drawn into my story and the mission I was on. Though I didn't realize it then, she became an integral part of our journey—a mentor and a significant voice of influence in our lives.

Dr. Brown introduced me to the concept of whole-child development, which expanded my perspective beyond Nathan's physical and academic growth to encompass his cognitive, social, emotional, psychological, and spiritual dimensions. I enrolled Nathan in swimming classes and Special Olympics with this broader outlook. Nathan wholeheartedly embraced both experiences, finding joy in them despite some distinctive aspects. For instance, he exclusively relied on one leg for kicking in his swimming lessons. During the Special Olympics, his greater strength in pushing compared to pulling led to a unique situation where he ended up being the only participant in the race going backward in his wheelchair.

Dr. Brown also played an essential role in motivating me to write my first book. She believed that doing so would create a platform for educating, inspiring, and advocating, ultimately fostering positive change and a deeper appreciation for both the challenges and strengths of individuals with disabilities.

EMPOWERING SPEECH AND CONNECTION

I had almost given up on speech services for Nathan. By the time he turned twelve, he had undergone three speech evaluations in the US, receiving only about ten hours of therapy, with the last session occurring when he was just five years old. My encounter with Erin Mercer in 2016 was serendipitous. I had received a grant from a UK-based disability training agency to create a pilot model for a Rehabilitation Aides program aimed at supporting children with multiple disabilities in a local children's home. Erin applied for the speech therapist position, and like Senta, from the moment we met, I could see her compassion, empathy, and expertise shine through.

Erin seamlessly integrates her clinical expertise, unwavering empathy, and a deeply client-centered approach to empower individuals in enhancing their communication and swallowing capabilities, thus elevating their overall quality of life. I distinctly recall her inaugural encounter with a young child in Jamaica, a stark departure from the traditional clinical setting we were accustomed to, where clinicians typically remained behind imposing desks during therapy sessions. Instead, Erin chose to join the child on a play mat, the child being around five years old. By the end of the session, the child emerged from the room with a radiant smile, exclaiming, "Mommy, this wasn't therapy; it was play!"

Another remarkable trait of Erin that continues to inspire me is her remarkable ability to code switch, adapting her communication style to ensure her audience feels heard, respected, and empowered. Whenever she arrived in Jamaica for our brief yet intensive "speech clinics," Erin tirelessly dedicated herself to the cause, working diligently from the moment her plane touched down until the time of her departure. She recognized the urgent need for speech therapy services for a significant number of children in the region.

Erin's impact extended even further. She played a pivotal role in helping Nathan access his first augmented communication device when he was twelve. She provided training in the use of his device to my family and all the teachers at Nathan's school. This kindness began to unlock his expressive communication skills, giving him a voice. She has been a reliable sounding board when I encountered frustration and needed to talk through solutions.

Our journey together transcended the boundaries of mere collaboration, evolving into a beautiful friendship. Erin has been a pillar of support for me in numerous ways; I will share more about this in upcoming chapters. I deeply value her friendship, professional humility, and how she generously pours into the lives of others in service to God.

Before wrapping up this chapter, I want to share the stories of two remarkable individuals: Elaine, whom I affectionately refer to as my self-leader coach, and Karaine, one of my most ardent cheerleaders. My initial encounter with Elaine occurred almost a decade before when she conducted a self-leadership workshop for my corporate team. However, we lost touch over time. In 2011, while fervently praying for someone to moderate a national disability workshop I was hosting, fate intervened. I unexpectedly ran into Elaine, and as we caught up, she expressed her keen interest in supporting my work. Just like that, we rekindled our connection. With just a week's notice, she graciously agreed to moderate the event's opening day pro bono, and it felt like a match made in heaven.

Elaine played an instrumental role in helping me establish a clear boundary between myself and the Nathan Ebanks Foundation. I struggled to distinguish between my personal identity and the identity of the foundation. She graciously opened her heart and home to me, and for several years, we convened under the shade of a magnificent lignum vitae tree in her lush tropical gardens. She poured her wisdom into me, constantly reminding me of my success as a marketer before Nathan and the foundation became focal points in my life. She offered counseling, coaching, untiring support, and a safe space for me to undertake the rebuilding of my identity and confidence.

Elaine's voice serves as a constant reminder of my commitment to the vision of serving others. She emphasizes that our purpose on this planet is to be a blessing to those around us. Under her guidance, I have refined my abilities in active listening, upholding professional boundaries, and embracing authenticity. I deeply admire her talent for bridging the gap between the practical and spiritual realms. She has consistently been an outstanding sounding board, offering a wealth of tools and strategies that have empowered me to surmount obstacles and foster personal and spiritual growth.

Another significant contributor to my support and personal growth is Karaine Smith Holness. Although we were in the same Jamaican high school and graduating class, we never met. I joined the graduating class alumni group on social media more than two years later. Karaine came across my story and reached out to me. It was during one of my lowest moments, and our conversation flowed as if we were old friends. She generously offered me the gift of her attentive and compassionate listening.

Karaine called me weekly for about a month, creating a safe space for me to release some of the burdens I was carrying. She also took action in her community in Connecticut, rallying support for the Nathan Ebanks Foundation's work. She became a passionate advocate for our cause, and thanks to her efforts, we were able to host many programs giving children access to speech therapy evaluations and other resources.

One of the most touching memories I have from our conversations is how, during those moments when tears overwhelmed me, I could hear the emotion in her own voice as she listened. After the loss of Dawn, Karaine stepped into that void with remarkable intuition, always knowing precisely when to reach out and provide her support, lifting my spirits when I needed it most.

She introduced me and my work to the US almost a decade before my family and I would immigrate here. I fondly call her my connector because she carries our mission in her heart wherever she goes and doesn't shy away from sharing it with others. She effectively drew in the support of other alumni living in the US, and while some have moved on, each one has played a crucial role in my journey.

These journey companions of mine, Senta, Dawn, Elaine, Wendean, Lisa, Karaine, and Erin, are but some of the individuals who stepped into my story, affirming for me that the presence of others is essential for creating a nurturing and inclusive environment for families raising a child with disabilities. They have offered emotional, practical, and social support that helped enhance my well-being so that I can be useful to my family and the families I serve through the Nathan Ebanks Foundation.

TAKEAWAY

I included this chapter because I'm a firm believer in sharing the whole story. When outsiders look at my family, they might assume that Nathan's progress and identity are solely the result of our efforts. The age-old African proverb wisely reminds us, "It takes a village to raise a child." This saying underscores the notion that child-rearing and nurturing are collaborative efforts that involve the collective support of a community or network of individuals, extending beyond the role of parents and families alone. And when a child like Nathan confronts the distinctive challenges of a disability, that village metamorphoses into a multifaceted, interdisciplinary community, which, as my dear friend Senta aptly puts it, can be likened to a tribe.

I want to be clear about the enormity of what it has taken to raise this child, Nathan, this gift from God. As someone once told me, it was never God's intention that we go the path alone. He provided these rich, diverse individuals and professionals from various walks of life. I marvel at how this support unfolded from a local and international community who came into our lives because of Nathan. They didn't just extend a helping hand; they created a network of understanding, empathy, and advocacy.

In their presence, this journey against the odds felt less isolating, the obstacles more surmountable, and the accomplishments, more meaningful. Their active involvement reinforces my belief that no family should have to walk this path of raising a child with disabilities alone.

CHAPTER 20

TRUSTING IN GOD'S PLAN

Back to the Present

A gentle touch on my shoulder jolted me from the depths of my thoughts, pulling me back to the present—Saturday afternoon, April 8, 2023. I looked up to see my daughter, Jordanne, gazing at me with concern. "Mom, Mommy, are you okay?" she asked, her eyes reflecting her worry. For a brief moment, I didn't know where I was. Then I remembered—I was sitting in the ICU waiting room.

We were facing the third major medical event of Nathan's young life. He had been admitted the night before due to severe stomach pains and continuous vomiting. I had met with the doctor earlier, and he diagnosed him with an intestinal blockage, indicating the necessity of emergency surgery scheduled for that day. After they had taken him to radiology for tests and insertion of NG tubes to prepare for his treatment and surgery, I walked to the waiting room to await Jordanne's arrival.

Amidst the weightiness of the current situation, I was grateful to find a quiet place to wait. It let my mind wander back in time, retracing Nathan's incredible journey. Like a beautiful tapestry, I saw threads of courage, resilience, and unwavering determination forming its pattern. More importantly, I saw the hand of God with us in each challenge, guiding our steps to overcome the many obstacles stacked against him. I recalled the surgeon from his first significant health event shortly after birth gave him a fifty-fifty chance of surviving infancy. Yet, here we were; Nathan was eighteen and on the cusp of his nineteenth birthday. He had survived childhood.

I was also grateful for the encouragement I discovered as I scrolled through the book of Psalms on my phone. Psalm 77:11–12 (NIV) leaped out and seemed to whisper directly to my heart: "I will remember the deeds of the Lord; yes, I will remember your miracles of long ago. I will consider all your works and meditate on all your mighty deeds." At that moment, a realization washed over me—this was precisely what I was doing as I waited. The verses gained a deep and humbling resonance. They were yet another reminder that God was fully in control. Every trial we had faced, every valley we had journeyed through, was a thread woven into a vast tapestry, infused with purpose and embraced by grace.

I felt assured that although the reasons behind the current circumstances eluded me, Nathan would also overcome this trial. Because of God's inherent kindness and benevolence, I could find comfort in the certainty that His plans for us were marked by goodness. I felt ready to face whatever was ahead of us.

With this matter settled, I smiled and assured Jordanne everything was alright. In an unexpected turn, I discovered a genuine sense of tranquility as I sifted through my emotions. I was intrigued to observe the distinct contrast between my present state of composure and the tempest of emotions that nearly engulfed me during Nathan's initial days in the NICU after his birth. I marveled at how the passage of time had gradually fortified my resilience in the realm of raising a child with special needs. This journey gifted me with various coping mechanisms and insights that seasoned me to confront whatever adversities lay on the horizon. Equally important, it nurtured a deep connection between my faith and practical life, teaching me to seek and trust God in the ordinary moments of everyday existence.

A quick glance at my watch indicated it was time to head back, as Nathan should have returned to the room. I had been sitting in the lobby for a long time. As I linked my arm with Jordanne's, I was grateful she was there. Walking together, I could see how accustomed I had become to taking on these experiences on my own. It had become my automatic response, despite the significant shifts in our family dynamic since Nathan's birth— my older children were now young adults. I was thankful that this time, things were different. I was not alone spiritually and physically.

There Was No Early Warning Signs

Except for a singular episode of pneumonia at age two, Nathan's health had demonstrated remarkable resilience over the years. He had developed into one of the sturdiest individuals I had ever encountered. With time, occurrences of colds and the flu became increasingly rare. Even amidst our immigration to the United States at the peak of the COVID-19 pandemic, Nathan's susceptibility—tripled by his underlying disability—remained untouched. His consistently sound health had gradually shaped our new normal, lulling us into a false sense that his challenges were firmly in the past. So, this sudden health event caught us all off guard.

Nathan's growth and development have been remarkable since our move to the United States as Green Card permanent-resident immigrants in 2020. Our early concerns about his transition, considering he was sixteen at the time of our move and had recently lost his Grandpa Ebanks, were unfounded. He adapted more smoothly than the rest of us. While his school transition had many challenges, it was evident that the district and teachers were committed to working with him (and us). In fact, I learned that the teachers affectionately referred to him as "Nate the Great," and he was playfully dubbed the "mayor" of the school due to his popularity. And in return, he embraced school enthusiastically, eagerly boarding the school bus each day with a heart full of joy.

He was in his senior year, enjoying the rights and privileges of seniors, when the illness occurred. Just the day before Good Friday, Jordanne and I took him on a special outing to the shopping mall, an experience he relished. It allowed him to savor his favorite foods and indulge in one of his cherished pastimes—observing people. As we wandered through the mall, Nathan's radiant smile and unique "ello" (hello) vocalizations filled the air, instantly recognizable to those who knew him. His joyful interactions brightened the countenance of most people we passed.

We ended our mall excursion with a whimsical and endearing photo session starring Nathan and the Easter Bunny. The laughter and delight that bubbled from him were infectious, leaving him brimming with contentment as we returned home. When the vomiting started later that night, it didn't trigger alarm bells. After all, it had become a regular part of his life, something we were accustomed to. I sprang into action, giving him rehydration fluids, thinking it would help ease the situation. But as time passed, it became painfully clear that he couldn't hold anything down. The vomiting took on a more intense and forceful nature, and that's when my concern grew.

In a moment of uncertainty, I reached out to a friend who is a nurse. I needed advice. *Was this something that warranted a trip to the emergency room (ER)?* Her words echoed reassurance, "Keep doing what you're doing and observe him closely."

But as the night unfolded, none of us got much sleep. By morning, exhaustion was joined by heightened worry. Evidently, Nathan was not well; his cheerful countenance disappeared, and he seemed to be in pain, which was another concern as he had a high tolerance for pain. I knew it was time to seek help beyond our home's walls. I scheduled a virtual visit with the emergency doctor at his pediatrician's office. Together, we leaned toward the possibility of a stomach bug, and she prescribed anti-nausea medication. Her advice was to monitor him for another day or two and consider the ER if things didn't improve.

However, with the progression of the day, his condition rapidly deteriorated. He wasn't holding anything down—not even the prescribed medication or rehydration fluids. By early afternoon, he looked dehydrated; his skin was clammy, and he was writhing in pain and crying. It was then that that small inner voice, the constant companion since his birth, spoke with clarity, urgency, and insistence, telling me to take him to the ER. Having learned to trust my instinct when it came to him, I listened.

Robert was asleep after his night shift, Adrianne was at work, and Ryan was home on a Friday off. I shared my concern with him, and he agreed we needed to go immediately. I drove to the hospital affiliated with Nathan's pediatrician, passing another on my way. As I passed the first hospital, I noticed a sign: "Plenty of patient parking." Though it struck me, I knew the reason would become clear if it mattered.

Sure enough, at the intended hospital, parking was scarce. I circled for about twenty minutes, trying to stop temporarily for Ryan to take Nathan to the ER while I searched for parking. As Nathan's cries became louder, I gave up and returned to the hospital with plenty of patient parking space. Upon our arrival at the ER, the intake process was swift, and in under thirty minutes, he was situated in a bed, being set up with intravenous (IV) lines.

I felt a deep ache for him as I observed his evident distress while he lay in the hospital bed. My mind was still occupied with the notion of a potential stomach virus and dehydration as I responded to the intake questions, which involved recounting his medical history from my pregnancy onward. Throughout this process, I took comfort in the assumption that he might receive medication and fluids for rehydration, possibly leading to his discharge after a few hours. The notion that his condition could be serious had not yet entered my thoughts.

Subsequently, when the doctor disclosed the results following several X-rays and a CT scan, indicating a blockage in his intestine, a mix of thoughts raced through my mind. The doctor offered reassurance, explaining that while it might indeed be related to accumulated stool, something more serious could be at play. They emphasized the need for further tests, including an enema, to ascertain the exact nature of the issue. Despite the uncertainties, I initially found myself leaning toward stool accumulation. It had been quite some time since Nathan had experienced any significant health concerns, and the sudden onset of a severe illness seemed unlikely. With his occasional struggles with constipation in mind, the notion of stool accumulation felt more plausible and manageable.

After monitoring him throughout the night, the doctor shared their insights. There being no change in his condition, the only way forward was emergency surgery. During this discussion, the doctor also shared a crucial nugget of information: patients who had previously undergone abdominal surgeries or surgeries similar to Nathan's were more susceptible to such blockages. This disclosure left no room for uncertainty—Nathan's ongoing ordeal was undeniably a case of intestinal blockage.

The diagnosis hit me unexpectedly, but my innate "case manager" instinct kicked in. I swiftly switched into clinical mode, engaging with various healthcare professionals and technicians to grasp the situation thoroughly. This was crucial to accurately relay the unfolding events to our family group chat. Furthermore, as questions poured in from different family members via the chat, I seamlessly acted as the bridge between them and the medical team. This engagement kept me preoccupied, which was a welcome distraction so I wouldn't have to focus on what was rapidly unfolding.

PRE-SURGERY PREPARATIONS

As we approached Nathan's room, I saw he was back in his bed with a team of doctors. My pace quickened, and upon our entry, they turned their attention to us, verifying our identity before explaining the upcoming procedures. The surgeon assumed the lead, elaborating on the forthcoming course of action.

As I listened, I knew that after all these years, "someone still kept watch" over Nathan because the prompting of that still, small voice that urged me to take him into the ER had saved his life once again. I was grateful for the years of practice of listening to that voice that had built up my instincts because the doctor explained that if we had waited to take him in a day or two later, his condition might have been fatal.

Guiding us through the upcoming stages, the surgeon explained that the core issue of the blockage likely stemmed from a twisting of the intestines, disrupting blood flow and the normal movement of food, liquids, and waste. This provided insight into Nathan's ongoing abdominal discomfort and pain. The surgeon stressed the situation's urgency, highlighting that delaying the surgery could potentially lead to life-threatening complications.

In addition, he explained that the surgery would be done under general anesthesia. Depending on the nature and location of the blockage, they might choose to excise the obstructed part of the intestine (resection)[26] or conduct repairs to address the issue. He further stated that an intestinal anastomosis could be required to reconnect the healthy portions of the intestine.

He also touched on the potential for post-surgery complications. Still, my mind was fixed on proceeding with the surgery because I understood that not doing it wasn't a viable option. So, I signed the consent forms.

---

26 This procedure involves removing a portion of the intestines (small intestine or large intestine) due to various reasons such as disease, blockage, or injury. The remaining healthy segments of the intestines are then reconnected or attached to each other, as well as to the stomach or another part of the digestive tract.

Until that point, I had been effectively managing my emotions. However, my composed demeanor took a nosedive when the doctor brought up the do-not-resuscitate (DNR) order. As he elaborated, DNRs are medical directives indicating a person's choice to forego cardiopulmonary resuscitation (CPR) if a cardiac or respiratory arrest occurs during a medical procedure. The doctor emphasized that the hospital follows a protocol of resuscitation, and thus, patients are required by law to establish their preferred directive before undergoing any surgical procedures. This enables patients and their families to carefully deliberate on their preferences concerning such crucial decisions.

On the one hand, I appreciated their comprehensive communication on this matter. At the same time, I was uncertain whether I truly wanted to confront this information. It opened up a realm of consideration I wasn't quite prepared to delve into—the acknowledgment that there existed the potential for complications during or after the surgery.

He proceeded to underscore the potential outcomes of resuscitation during a critical event, outlining scenarios that ranged from the risk of sustaining brain damage to the potential of slipping into a coma—all of which could result in a diminished quality of life for the patient. It was substantial information to absorb all at once, especially as I fought to maintain composure while witnessing Nathan's evident discomfort.

This was the first time I had this type of discussion concerning Nathan or any family member, for that matter. As the doctor spoke, a sense of panic began to well up within me. I wanted to cover my ears rather than face this unsettling possibility that the outcome might not be what I wanted. Suddenly, it became hard to breathe, and I was startled by a gentle squeeze on my hand.

It was Jordanne, a welcome reminder that I wasn't alone in the moment.

"It's alright, Mom," she whispered. As if reading my thoughts, she continued. "He is not saying any of this will happen to Nathan. He is following the HIPAA regulations[27] (and the hospital policy), which mandates that patients be informed so they can exercise their right to choose." Upon hearing her words, a wave of relief washed over me, allowing me to finally catch my breath. As I endeavored to regain my emotional composure, Jordanne assumed control, directing inquiries toward the doctor. Her gentle hand resting on mine became a steadfast anchor, a continuous wellspring of comfort throughout the remainder of our conversation.

I was grateful that I didn't have to walk the path alone this time. I was also grateful to Jordanne for choosing to pursue a speech-language pathology course of study, giving her a clear understanding of hospital procedures like this one. As our conversation flowed, the medical team wrapped up their preparations, readying to transport Nathan to the operating room. To my surprise and relief, the doctor invited us to accompany him to the operating room, a practice not common back in Jamaica. This unexpected gesture brought a wave of comfort. Walking on either side of Nathan, we held his hands, offering our presence as a source of comfort and assurance. With each step, we reassured him that we would be there when he returned. I prayed silently, covering him, the doctors, and all who were part of this process.

Upon entering the outer room of the operating theater, the

---

27 The acronym "HIPAA" stands for the Health Insurance Portability and Accountability Act. It is a federal law enacted in the United States in 1996 to address several important aspects of healthcare, health insurance, and medical information security.

attending doctors offered a succinct outline of the procedure and its anticipated duration. They handed me additional consent forms for my signature. With that settled, Jordanne and I proceeded to the cafeteria to grab a meal while we awaited the surgery's completion. As we made our meal choices, I found myself drawing parallels between this experience and our first encounter with surgery. On that occasion, I was alone, with no chance to step away for refreshment during the wait. I also lacked the understanding of what to expect in terms of timing and outcomes. Equally important, Jordanne and I had the privilege of accompanying Nathan to the operating theater, reassuring me that he knew he was not alone. Although the surgery had not yet begun, it was evident that this time, things were noticeably better.

We had barely settled down to have our first meal of the day when my phone rang, and my heart skipped a beat upon seeing the hospital's name on the caller ID. Yet, the anxiety soon eased as one of the resident surgeons introduced himself and inquired about my location. I shared that I was in the cafeteria. He then disclosed that a crucial document still required my signature, and to my surprise, he generously offered to bring it to me so he would not disrupt my meal.

This was the very essence of redemption—a subtle yet profound transformation of both the circumstances and my own perspective. As I sat in the cafeteria, tightly gripping my phone, I couldn't help but marvel at how far we had come. The memories of Nathan's first hospitalization had been etched into my soul like scars, but they no longer held the power to paralyze me with fear.

The actions of these strangers, these dedicated medical practitioners, were indeed rewriting the narrative for me. They had become agents of healing, delicately tending to the wounds left by the traumas of the past. Their kindness, compassion, and how they treated Nathan not as a patient but as a person were like soothing balm into the persistent ache of those long past memories. It carried a gentle undercurrent of hope, much like a soft, reassuring whisper amid uncertainty. A soft chuckle escaped my lips as I glanced upward and softly murmured, "I see You, Lord. Yes, I truly see You. Thank You."

As we walked the long corridors on our way to the parking lot that evening, my gaze was drawn to a particular feature adorning the hospital walls. There, a multitude of frames displayed a treasure trove of information, encapsulating the very heart of the hospital—its identity, core values, guiding principles, and its declaration of commitment to patient care and the well-being of the community. One of these frames had the following words:

> We minister to the whole person, body, and spirit, preserving the dignity and sacredness of each life. We are pledged to the creation of an environment of mutual support among our employees, physicians, and volunteers and to the education and training of healthcare personnel.
>
> We are witnesses in our community to the highest ethical and moral principles in pursuit of excellence and patient safety.[28]

In that moment, it became evident that we were exactly where we were meant to be. The close proximity of this place to our home and its alignment with our faith showed that God had or-

28 "Saint Peter's University Hospital," Saint Peter's Healthcare System, accessed November 15, 2023, https://staging.saintpetershcs.com/Locations/Saint-Peter-s-University-Hospital.

chestrated this deeply redemptive experience, for which I was grateful.

TAKEAWAY

Until this recent experience, I hadn't fully grasped the enduring trauma I carried from past hospital care for Nathan. I had believed time, forgiveness, acceptance, and releasing the past had sufficed, thinking I had conquered the fear those memories had instilled. However, all those emotions and anxieties came flooding back unexpectedly. It took a new, compassionate, positive encounter to finally rewrite those old memories. The care and kindness we experienced this third time around made me realize that I had been shouldering this trauma for far too long.

It underscored that the journey of recovery from trauma or challenging experiences doesn't typically follow a straightforward, upward trajectory; instead, it often proves to be a complex process. Healing can encompass highs and lows, setbacks, and unforeseen triggers that resurface painful emotions or memories, sometimes catching individuals off guard just when they thought they had moved past a particular issue. In our experience, I came to realize that the healing process is highly individualized and subject to variation. It became evident that having a supportive network and compassionate healthcare practitioners can significantly facilitate and accelerate the healing journey.

CHAPTER 21

WHEN THE PIECES FALL IN PLACE

Finding Purpose in Advocacy

After the surgery, Nathan was transported back to his room in the ICU. This time, his wound, which extended vertically from his chest to his lower abdomen, was held together with staples instead of a horizontally wrapped bandage around his midsection. He had also returned with NG tubes in both nostrils, one of which was actively draining bile from his stomach into a large jar. Seeing him in this condition was heart-wrenching, realizing he hadn't done anything to deserve the challenges life had thrown at him.

As the surgeon concluded his examination, I inquired about the next steps. He replied, "Now, we must wait. Nathan's body will determine our course of action from here." And just like that, I found myself in yet another waiting period.

It's truly amazing how much one's mind can wander during these seemingly endless waiting spells. As I sat by Nathan's side during the daytime, my mind drifted to the countless parents I've known whose children had to endure multiple surgeries at such a young age. I remembered another child named Nathan, a former classmate of my son in Jamaica, who had a rare chromosome disorder. When I spoke to his mother back then, I was shocked to learn that he had already undergone six major surgeries before his seventh birthday. Sitting by my Nathan's bedside now, I could truly empathize with what that parent and her family must have endured with their beloved son. As I contemplated this situation and the countless parents who had walked, are walking, and will walk a similar path, I couldn't deny that no matter how frequently it happens, the journey never becomes any easier.

Thankfully, this time, I didn't have to face this trial alone as I did in the past. Aside from our now-grown children, technology, through the family group chat, brought my family right into the room with me. Our conversations flowed, allowing us to seamlessly share information, support, encourage, laugh, and pray together. My smartphone gave me unrestricted access to the internet, allowing me to research and gather information to understand better how I could contribute to his care and recovery, as well as what to expect in the future so that I could plan accordingly. Managing my social media pages also kept me connected to our global community's numerous prayers and well-wishes, which lifted my spirits.

I thought back to the surgeon's post-surgery explanation regarding Nathan's condition, a volvulus. This condition occurs when a segment of the intestine twists around itself and the mesentery, the supportive tissue surrounding it, resulting in a significant bowel obstruction.[29] In Nathan's case, this twist led to

---

29 Kritika Krishnamurthy, Siba El Hussein, and Yumna Omarzai, "The lethal twist - a story of unspoken pain: small intestinal volvulus in cerebral palsy," Autopsy and Case Reports 8, no. 3,

the unfortunate consequence of approximately nine inches of his intestines becoming nonviable due to inadequate blood supply. Consequently, surgical removal was necessary, resulting in the loss of this portion of the intestine.

To complicate matters, the remaining intestine was too short for a straightforward reconnection. To address this issue, the medical team opted for a specialized procedure known as an "intestinal bypass" or "intestinal diversion." This procedure was employed to create a connection between the remaining intestine and his stomach.[30]

Initially, the intricacies and implications of this situation were unclear to me. Fortunately, the surgeon provided a more detailed explanation. He explained that internal organs often enter a kind of "sleep mode" when subjected to surgical manipulation, as was the case with Nathan. This meant that Nathan's body would require time for healing and for these organs to "awaken" from this state. The surgeon estimated that this recovery could span ten to fourteen days. During this period, there was an increased vulnerability to potential post-surgery complications, necessitating close monitoring. Furthermore, while Nathan's stomach was healing, they needed to install a peripherally inserted central catheter (PICC)[31] line to nourish him intravenously.

I contemplated the similarities between his first surgery, CDH, when he was only three days old and this recent intestinal

https://doi.org/10.4322/acr.2018.037.

30 Francesk Mulita and Saran Lotfollahzadeh, "Intestinal stoma," National Library of Medicine, June 3, 2023, https://www.ncbi.nlm.nih.gov/books/NBK565910.
31 A PICC line (peripherally inserted central catheter) is a long, thin tube that is inserted into a vein in the arm and advanced until the tip reaches a larger vein near the heart, used to provide long-term intravenous (IV) access for various medical purposes, such as delivering medications, fluids, and nutrients.

obstruction surgery eighteen years later. While there are notable distinctions in the surgical approaches and the medical conditions they addressed, I couldn't help but observe their striking similarities: both procedures required general anesthesia and demanded vigilant postoperative monitoring due to potential complications such as infection, bleeding, or anesthesia-related issues. Furthermore, both surgeries had a profound impact on his internal organs, necessitating a period of rest for his stomach.

It was a sobering realization, but at the same time, this most recent surgery provided me with a deeper understanding of the first one, if that makes sense. Instinctively, I grasped the significance of it all. Additionally, I gained a clearer sense of my role: to be his advocate in the hospital, to assure him that he was not alone, to stay in prayer, and to keep a positive outlook.

I also found myself in a state of reflective gratitude, realizing that if this health event had happened while we were still living in Jamaica or during the peak of the COVID-19 pandemic, Nathan's outcome might have been vastly different.

While I watched over Nathan in the hospital room, I gradually linked our earlier experiences in the initial phases of our journey with our present circumstances. It felt like a sudden realization, as if a light bulb had turned on. The connection had escaped me until that moment, and upon its recognition, I realized that our past had indeed prepared and equipped us for the present. My heart swelled with gratitude and thankfulness. I came to realize that the countless years we spent in medical facilities in Jamaica and the USA, the hundreds of hours spent with therapists and various specialists, and his earlier hospitalizations had provided me with an intuitive understanding of the essential elements of his medical history that is important, storing this knowledge in the forefront of my memory. This familiarity made it easier for me to provide the necessary information efficiently and responsively in various situations. Furthermore, I recognized that my extensive advocacy experience in Jamaica and within the US education system had honed my abilities as a healthcare advocate. This, in turn, enabled me to communicate with the present healthcare personnel confidently and calmly and better understand Nathan and the characteristics of his disability under different stresses. This, in turn, helped me manage my worries and alleviate stress.

I also observed a significant boost in my confidence when conversing with the different healthcare professionals. Unlike in the past, I no longer hesitated to ask for explanations in simpler terms, often lightening the mood with a comment like, "Could you break that down for me in everyday language?" This approach often elicited smiles or chuckles from the medical team, signaling my candid acknowledgment of my limited understanding of certain medical terms.

I reflected on how tongue-tied I used to feel, uncertain about my role and significance in the medical context. There used to be a sense of embarrassment stemming from what I didn't know or couldn't pronounce. I vividly recalled my initial struggle with pronouncing "cerebral palsy (*seh-*'ree-*bruhl* 'pah-*zee*)" after we received the diagnosis. It took me about a year to master it without stumbling over my words. Now, I find it somewhat amusing when even professionals struggle with its pronunciation because my experience has shown that, aside from being a skilled linguist, those who pronounce it effortlessly often have lived or working experience with this condition.

Indeed, as I reflected during that waiting period, I became acutely aware of the abundant blessings and gifts that our past had bestowed upon us. My heart brimmed with gratitude and thanksgiving because, for the first time, I could unmistakably trace the hand of God from the very beginning of our journey to this precise moment. It was a revelation that went beyond mere realization; it was a deep understanding that our experiences were shaping a purposeful path.

I now saw how advocating for Nathan and others in similar situations was not only a way to navigate the challenges of his condition but also a means of discovering purpose, making a positive impact, and contributing to the creation of a more inclusive and compassionate world for individuals with disabilities.

FOSTERING RESILIENCE

One crucial lesson I've learned through advocacy is the necessity of unswerving resilience when confronted with setbacks and obstacles. Successfully navigating these challenges, particularly when advocating for a child with a disability, can lead to remarkable outcomes, including personal growth and accomplishment.

As I sat there, observing the nurses going about their tasks and listening to the rhythmic cadence of my son's breathing, I couldn't help but reflect on how our past challenges didn't block our path as I had thought but acted as catalysts for personal development.

Looking back, I realized that if the surgeon during my child's first surgery had provided me with the same level of information I received during this second experience, it might have overwhelmed me with an excess of early knowledge about the challenges and difficulties of raising a child with disabilities. While knowledge is unquestionably valuable, an inundation of information at an early stage can lead to excessive anxiety and stress. Excessive knowledge could have clouded my perspective and hindered the natural bonding process with my child.

However, in His infinite wisdom, God understood the delicate dance required to strike a balance between staying informed and embracing hope. Given how things unfolded, we were allowed to concentrate on nurturing our child's strengths, rejoicing in his milestones, and allowing his distinctive development to unfold organically. As I've discovered, the journey continually evolves, and achieving this equilibrium at every stage guarantees a more enriching and fulfilling experience for both our family and Nathan.

Indeed, Jesus imparts several fundamental lessons on this matter through His teachings. He emphasizes the idea that the path of faith is not devoid of challenges and hardships. He urges His followers to demonstrate endurance and perseverance when confronted with trials and tribulations, consistently advocating for the refusal to surrender, even in the face of adversity.

Jesus also underscores the importance of faith and unwavering trust in God throughout His teachings. He motivates His disciples to place their trust in God's providence and maintain their faith, even amid uncertainty. Additionally, He champions the concept of fostering a sense of community and mutual support among believers. Frequently, He stresses the significance of displaying love for one another, bearing each other's burdens, and offering assistance to fellow travelers on this journey.

Furthermore, Jesus imparts wisdom about resilience and overcoming obstacles, emphasizing that faith and prayer can surmount challenges and barriers. He shares stories and examples of individuals who encountered adversity but drew strength from their faith to overcome it. In that hospital room, I could clearly see all of these lessons springing to life in our journey of raising Nathan, this precious gift from God.

STRENGTH OF THE TRIBE

It was miraculous how all the pieces moved in place to wrap around Nathan after that. It was as if everything that happened to our family before had been rehearsed for this moment. Robert called out from work to take over the night shift from Jordanne and me. Adrianne and Ryan came with him to the hospital to see Nathan and bring some of his favorite toys to make him more comfortable. I stood there, listening as they worked out a schedule of who would come when to ensure that I was never alone and that someone was with him around the clock.

The hospital's team was simply amazing. Each specialist who came to see us took the time to explain in language that we understood their process and what we could expect over the days following the surgery. The nurses were particularly supportive, empathetic, and compassionate.

I thought back to the wise words of that kind older matron the day I took Nathan home after he survived his first surgery. "Let your baby be around his siblings. Teach them to play with him and care for him. Make his life in your family 'normal,' don't keep him from them." Little did I realize back then just how impactful those seemingly simple words would be. It was about fostering a sense of togetherness and unity, ultimately becoming a cornerstone of our family's resilience as we forged our close-knit bond, building our inner tribe.

As we journeyed home that evening, I whispered quietly, "Thank You, God, for bestowing me the precious gift of Nathan, my children, and my family. I am grateful for the wisdom of Your words in Proverbs 22:6 (NKJV), which instructs us, 'Train up a child in the way he should go: and when he is old, he will not depart from it.' Our circumstances are a living testament to the principles found in this scripture."

TAKEAWAY

The central message of this chapter underscores the transformative power of our life experiences. I've realized that nothing in our lives is wasted, no matter how seemingly insignificant. Everything has a way of working together, as life experiences act as valuable educators, offering fresh perspectives and invaluable insights that play a pivotal role in shaping our personal growth, enhancing decision-making, and strengthening relationships. These experiences also contribute to our resilience and overall well-being, providing valuable insights that can lead to a more meaningful and fulfilling life. In our case, it also underscored our resilience and adaptability in the face of formidable challenges, reinforcing our inner strength. Additionally, it unveiled the interconnectedness of our life experiences, illustrating how they contribute to our overarching life journey.

This was when it finally dawned on me. Our journey in raising Nathan was never about merely surviving (the destination). It was about thriving and blooming where we were planted. It was about growing to become wiser, true versions of ourselves (as human beings made in the image and likeness of God). Through these firsthand experiences, we learned profound lessons in faith, tenacity, empathy, and the enduring strength that resides within us. For, as we discovered, when we are firmly rooted in God, we can live meaningful, compelling, and purposeful lives filled with joy, love, and gratitude. I learned that, together with God, we are undaunted.

CHAPTER 22

SAME STORY, DIFFERENT PERSPECTIVE: ROBERT'S ACCOUNT

With Nathan in the hospital, the usual busyness of my days came to an abrupt halt. It dawned on me that, over the years, our lives had been significantly molded to accommodate Nathan's ever-changing needs.

We had become a tightly-knit unit when it came to Nathan's care and well-being. Our ability to adapt to the evolving demands of his condition had become second nature. From the very beginning, we approached decision-making for him as a united family, methodically considering and planning each step to ensure his accessibility, mobility, and support. Spontaneity became a luxury we willingly relinquished early on. Whether it was a simple overnight trip or any other outing, every aspect of our movements—

leaving home, safely transporting, feeding, entertaining, bathing, and putting Nathan to sleep—had to be meticulously planned. This practice transformed us into a resilient and cohesive team.

In the initial days following the surgery, it was difficult to see him lying in the hospital bed, still and unanimated, which was unusual. With his dyskinetic cerebral palsy, Nathan's body is typically in constant motion, even when asleep. When he's awake, his presence is unmistakably big. He engages us with his distinctive "ello" (hello) sounds as we pass by, calls our attention with unique sounds, and actively participates in whatever he's watching—be it animated fights with characters in his favorite shows or enthusiastically joining in praise and worship during our streamed church services.

Returning to an empty apartment each night was emotionally challenging. Stepping inside or waking up in the morning and not seeing his wheelchair tugged at my emotions. I hadn't realized just how much space he filled in our home. But everywhere I looked, there he was—baby photos, milestones like his high school senior pictures on the wall, soft toys tucked away in corners of the room, and even turning on the "big" TV, dubbed as "Nathan's TV," were constant reminders. The apartment felt unusually quiet, as if it, too, recognized his absence. With so much more time on my hands, I felt disoriented.

Nonetheless, I was pleased that I managed to maintain my emotional composure. I was active in the personal aspects of his care at the hospital despite the nurses' assurance that it wasn't necessary. I read to him, engaged in conversations, and recited scriptures and affirmations to uplift his spirits. Simultaneously, I kept open communication with my family and friends, posted regular updates on social media, promptly responded to comments, offered prayers, expressed gratitude to God, and consistently maintained a positive and upbeat demeanor.

Then, on the fifth day, the emotional floodgates finally gave way. As I prepared to go to the hospital that morning, I inadvertently moved some clothing on the small sofa in my bedroom, causing a single foot of Nathan's sock to tumble to the floor. I didn't know it was there, but the trigger shattered the emotional dam I had carefully held in check. Tears welled up and then spilled uncontrollably, as if from the very core of my being. But this time, it felt different. There was no fear or anxiety that had plagued me in the past. I harbored no doubt about his recovery; it was a cathartic release, a way for me to let go of the pent-up emotions, stress, and tension that had built up inside.

I allowed the emotions to flow freely, tears streaming down my face for nearly half an hour until I felt emotionally drained. Afterward, I gathered myself, had breakfast, and made my way to the hospital. As I stepped out, I carried with me a profound lightness and a renewed sense of hope that had been missing for days.

Later that day, I shared this experience with Robert and my older children through our family group chat. It opened the door for them to express their emotions and share how this event impacted them. While I had always been aware of the deep love that Nathan's siblings and Robert had for him, in the past, I had never considered their perspectives on our shared journey.

The first and last time I did a check-in with each family member was back in 2018 during the research stage for my book *How to Cope: Parenting a Child with Special Needs*.[32] However, that day, as I read their comments in the group chat, it occurred to me

32 Christine Staple Ebanks, How to Cope: Parenting a Child with Special Needs (Kingston, Jamaica: Bala Press, 2018).

how much more mature and established they all were, signaling that it was a good time to do another check-in.

Their perspective on our shared experience was so revelatory, instructive, and moving that I felt compelled to include their voices in this book. It became clear that sharing only my side of the story would be telling just half of it. I have dedicated this and the next three chapters to them. Here is what they had to say.

ROBERT

The Early Days

Raising Nathan has become less difficult as the years go by. I can remember, after hearing the diagnosis of congenital diaphragmatic hernia when Christine was still pregnant with him, I had a mental picture of a child in a wheelchair. I spoke with the Lord quietly in my heart, telling Him I would not abandon my son but that I'd be there for him, no matter what. Having had that talk with God, I basically prepared myself mentally and emotionally for whatever would come.

However, as the pregnancy progressed, I never really thought about the diagnosis again. My focus shifted, and my sole concern was for my wife, Christine, and her well-being. My attention was centered on helping her to get through the pregnancy safely.

I remember when Nathan was born and had to be incubated in the hospital for some time. For his entire hospitalization, I ran on pure adrenaline, sitting with him each night after my MBA classes into the wee hours of the morning. Then, I would return home, snatch what little sleep I could, and wake up a few hours later to prepare his siblings, take them to school, and head to work.

I remember how difficult it was sitting with him during these visits. I couldn't touch him because he was in a sealed incubator. Instead, I watched over him and sang to him. It was a truly trying time, especially since I saw many babies die during his stay. I watched other fathers suffer emotional breakdowns as they visited their children. They left the day before, only to be told the child had passed away. I was sorry for their pain, but I could only pray that my baby, Nathan, would survive. And thanks be to God, he did!

When we received the cerebral palsy (CP) diagnosis, the image of a child in a wheelchair resurfaced in my mind. But nothing I imagined could have adequately prepared me for the reality of its impact on his life and ours. At the time, I had naively believed that he could lead a "normal" life despite his disability. Only recently did I confess to Christine how thankful I am that I didn't know then what I know now. If I had been aware of the challenges and limitations my son would face and the sometimes overwhelming impact it would have on all our lives, I honestly don't know if I would have had the same level of confidence back then to move forward.

A Father's Heart

People often ask me how I cope with the knowledge that my son has been permanently disabled since infancy and will always need support for his daily living. My response is straightforward: Nathan is my son, and I love him unconditionally. His presence in my life has brought about positive changes. When he smiles at me, it's impossible not to reciprocate with a smile. He's quite the "ladies' man" and possesses more charm and "game" than I could ever hope to have.

Of course, the flip side of all this is that I do look at children who are Nathan's age and see them doing age-appropriate things, and I feel sad because Nathan will never (Hope says, "Never say never") be able to do those things. For instance, his graduation from high school this past June (2023). It was tough to see him with his peers, knowing they were heading to college and Nathan was not. I am happy for them, but this also reflects another thing Nathan will never get to do.

But at the same time, when I look at my son, I see a brilliant kid. He is smart and intuitive. I remember one time when he was about four or five. We were lying on the carpet at home, and I used my body to block him from leaving a safe space to go toward the staircase. I watched him roll back and forth, and then, like a seasoned athlete, he flipped his body, bounced on the carpet, and vaulted over me to get to the other side. I was stunned, amazed, and proud all the same time.

I am always amazed how, with his limited range of motion, he created basic signs to communicate with us, many of which we still use today and which are now incorporated in his school's communication plan with him. Of course, he taught us his signs for "hungry," "thirsty," or which channel he wanted to watch on TV. He has also incorporated a few actual sign language patterns to help communicate. He has so many abilities and great qualities wrapped up in him that I wish others would take the time to get to know him. He brings so much joy to my life.

Another area that was a struggle for me was coming to terms with the knowledge that my son would never be able to play physical sports, such as football and basketball (some of my favorites), or that he may never become the physicist I wanted to be. Like my wife, Christine, I let go of *my* dreams for Nathan. I have learned instead to choose and expect God's best for him. He is a warrior and an overcomer; his life tells the tale and makes a difference for others.

My Coping Mechanisms

As a Christian familiar with the Bible, I knew of the word "palsy" but did not quite know what the illness was, except that it was only through the power of Jesus that the sick man was healed of this "palsy." That was all the information I had when Nathan was diagnosed, but I didn't know what to do, where to go, or what to look out for.

But, unlike Christine, my coping mechanisms were different. I didn't feel denial, anger, or grief. My main thought was, "This is my son, and his diagnosis is what it is." But I did fall into depression. I felt lost because I didn't know what to do, where to turn, or how to help him. I felt powerless as I watched my wife fall apart many times as she struggled to find answers.

My wife and I share a common faith in the Lord and depend on Him to take us through even the most difficult circumstances. However, despite this faith, my wife is the emotional one. She gets her release through crying, praying, talking, advocating, and writing. I, on the other hand, deal with it quietly and privately. I watched TV, read, browsed bookstores, took "alone time" on long car rides, and played football (soccer). I simply did physical things that occupied my mind and kept me from thinking and dwelling on my circumstances.

For years, I kept everything locked up inside. I never spoke to anyone other than my wife about how I felt and how I was coping. And even then, she was the one who usually initiated the conversation. When I do talk with her about my feelings, I stay on the surface of things. Often, our conversations end with me saying, "I am not focused on anything other than the love for my family and my commitment to just do what I have to do." While I know she would often like me to be more open, the truth is that this is where I can cope because anything deeper becomes over-whelming.

Another difference between my wife and me is that she looks at things in the "here and now"—handling Nathan's appoint-ments, seeking therapy interventions, dealing with his schooling, managing his aide, and daily care. I, on the other hand, see the "yesterday," the "today," and the "future" in the "here and now." For example, I worry about the day Nathan dies. I want to be there with him when that time comes. I have even researched the average lifespan of individuals with cerebral palsy. My wife, on the other hand, finds this morbid and doesn't like to talk about it. She prefers to remain hopeful and deal with things as they come.

But this is a recurring topic for me. Sometimes, I worry about who will take care of Nathan and help Christine if I die before him or if I get sick and cannot care for him. I don't want him to be a burden to the lives of his siblings, as I love the relationship between them.

Another question I get asked often is if I ever feel over-whelmed with the day-to-day living with Nathan. I must admit that I don't get overwhelmed with his personal care, but I do get overwhelmed when it feels like everyone in the household wants me to do many different things simultaneously. At times, I feel physically and emotionally tired. I watch my body gain weight, but I do not have the time or energy to work out. This makes me worry more about how I will remain healthy enough to continue looking after him as we all age. Despite this, I work hard to maintain balance in my life the best way I can. As Christine often reminds me, we were never given a manual on how to live this life we have been given. All we can do is to do the best we can.

I must confess, though, that one of the things that continues to anger me is the lack of accessibility and needed services. For example, when we lived in Jamaica, because of limited government support, the full burden of the cost of daily living, health care, and educational services for Nathan fell to our family. It was often challenging to fit everything into our monthly budget. In addition, health insurance in Jamaica did not cover the available services he needed. For example, Nathan needed a caregiver to go to school with him. We needed someone to help us at home, especially when everyone was out and Christine was home alone with Nathan. These costs came out of my monthly salary. His school fees, adaptive aides, and therapies were all our responsibility. At the end of the day, it added up!

The Blessings of Nathan

Reflecting on where we started and where I am now, I know I am more self-aware, better informed, and empowered to help Nathan. Before Nathan, I never gave disabilities a thought or invested any real interest in the subject. At that time, individuals with disabilities, children or adults, occupied very little space in my consciousness. But Nathan forced me to sit up, take notice, and get involved. I thank God for that.

As the years go by, I have released some of this fear. For instance, I used to worry about him not being able to enjoy his life or experience independence. Today, I have learned to see his joy as he navigates his life and participates in experiences as best as possible. Yes, seeing him in pain or being excluded still pains me. But I know he is a remarkably resilient young man, highly favored by God and blessed beyond measure. I know he holds the memories of happy times from his reactions when we look at home videos or photos. What more could I ask for as a father?

Living in the United States has truly been a blessing for Nathan and our family. Now, he has access to many of the essential services he needs, and I happily drive him to various therapies and appointments. Though it has only been three years since we immigrated here, I have witnessed remarkable improvements in him overall. However, I do notice that we still face challenges in accessing all the services he needs, with some having long waitlists. For instance, he has been on the clinical speech therapy waitlist for the last three years. But I am grateful that he gets some speech services through the school system.

Despite these hurdles, many aspects of his life have become more manageable. Take, for example, his medical emergency this past April 2023—a severe intestinal blockage. Surprisingly, it felt less overwhelming and easier to navigate than his previous hospitalizations in Jamaica.

When I look at my son today and how he is thriving and the opportunities he now has, I can't help but feel some degree of sadness when I think how different his life might have been if he had this level of access from the start. It makes me empathize even more with the children and families in my birth country who will never have this level of access. It also makes me appreciate more the privileges and blessings we have today.

Indeed, despite some progress, there is still work to be done in the US to provide more comprehensive support for families with children with special needs. While services are available, we often travel great distances for them. The ongoing juggling act of managing numerous clinical services, medical and dental appointments, school engagements, and daily living activities leaves us with minimal downtime. As a result, finding the time for regular exercise continues to be an enduring challenge.

Another big ticket concern is that as I grow older, I've noticed that lifting Nathan has become more demanding, particularly when it comes to activities such as carrying him upstairs. This is largely due to me physically slowing down and his substantial growth, as he now stands at a height of five feet nine inches (and is still growing). It often amuses Nathan to see me struggle when I transition him from his wheelchair to bed or to the bath. Although he helps Christine in these transitions, he tends to go limp when I lift him. Nonetheless, I have come to accept these physical challenges as an integral part of our extraordinary journey with our son.

Through it all, my faith continues to be my primary coping mechanism. Like my wife, my journey with Nathan has grown my faith and made it more practical. I don't really have close friends, so when I need comfort or am frustrated, there are several Bible verses that I turn to. One comes from 2 Corinthians 12:9 (NKJV), "My grace is sufficient for you, for My strength is made perfect in weakness." Upon that truth, I rely. Upon that truth, I release all my issues and concerns. Upon that truth, I focus not on my son's "dis-ability" but instead, as my wife encourages, on appreciating the gift that he is. My coping mechanism is powered only by Christ's strength, moving in on my weakness.

My wife and family are also great sources of blessings, comfort, and strength. Christine has a way of drawing me out and knowing when and how to pray for me even when I can't find the words to express my feelings. These help me to take limitations in strides with humility and grace.

In addition, these limitations have "cut me down to size" and pruned me of my "ego" that did not serve me well. I have learned (and am still learning) to "let go and let God!" And in that space, I am strong and can cope with any and everything that comes my way because, as I am learning, "His grace *is* sufficient" for me.

TAKEAWAY

This chapter underscores the significance of my husband Robert's perspective on our journey with Nathan. His viewpoint contributes a unique layer of understanding to our narrative, challenging me to expand my thinking beyond the immediate moment and consider how he processes our shared journey.

Throughout this book, I have candidly shared my own thoughts and emotions. However, it's essential to acknowledge that our journey isn't exclusively mine to narrate; it is a collective partnership involving God, our family, and the broader community of helpers and supporters. While I carry the primary caregiving responsibilities and serve as an advocate for Nathan, Robert, my other children, and our extended family and friends also play equally significant roles. Moreover, I appreciate how Robert's testimony underscores the lesson of the power of being equally yoked.

CHAPTER 23

SAME STORY, DIFFERENT PERSPECTIVE: ADRIANNE'S ACCOUNT

As I've mentioned before, in the early stages of raising Nathan, my focus was primarily on attending to my older children's physical needs. Little did I realize the profound emotional and psychological toll Nathan's situation was taking on them. Surprisingly, none of the medical or clinical specialists we encountered ever inquired about their well-being or how they were coping, leaving me unaware that I should have been checking in on them.

Looking back, I deeply wish I had possessed the knowledge I do now about the impact of a sibling's disability on other children within the family. Knowing what I know today, I would have undoubtedly approached things differently.

Remarkably, my daughter Adrianne rose to the occasion in this regard. She was only nine years old when Nathan was first diagnosed with CP, but she willingly became the pillar of support for her younger siblings, Ryan (seven) and Jordanne (five). They turned to her with their questions, seeking solace, and somehow, she found ways to simplify and explain things to them.

As the years went by, I observed that Ryan and Jordanne continued to look up to her. Ryan and Jordanne consistently place a high level of trust in Adrianne's words and guidance. There are even instances when Robert or I provide them with an answer, and they seek Adrianne's confirmation. She has, in fact, even assumed a role akin to a second mother for Nathan. Here's how that all unfolded.

ADRIANNE

The Early Days

I was eight years old when Nathan was born. Although my memory as a young child is limited, I do remember my mom's pregnancies and her pregnancy with Nathan. Being the firstborn, I welcomed my new siblings with joy and anticipation. My mom and dad had prepared me for what it would be like to have another sibling. So, I had the same expectations as Nathan for what would come. And I was really hoping that Nathan would be a girl! But alas, I had to come to terms with Nathan being a boy, as I realized that I was just happy to know we were having a new baby.

As the firstborn, the experience of welcoming a new sibling wasn't new to me. I had already done it twice before with Ryan and then Jordanne. However, I was much younger during those times: just twenty-two months old when Ryan was born and four years old when Jordanne came along. It was different with Nathan because I was seven and had a better concept of having a new baby to play with.

But like Ryan and Jordanne, I had a limited understanding of time and thought it was taking too long for the baby to be born. Mom and Dad brought us a children's book about pregnancy to ease our impatience. This remarkable 3D book vividly illustrated the fetus' development at various stages and explained the process in language tailored to our understanding. Oh, how we spent many happy hours every day eagerly exploring its pages and discussing what was happening from our perspectives. This helped to calm my worry as I could now see the different stages the baby was in.

I remember when the false alarms started. Dad would wake us late at night, saying our grandparents were there to pick us up as he had to rush Mommy to the hospital. This happened several times, and I didn't know what to expect each time. But Dad would come and get us and take us home. Several times, Mom didn't come home from the hospital right away. Other times, she would be home when we got there.

I wasn't sure what to expect the last time she was rushed to the hospital. I thought it was just another "false alarm." Because she was taken there in the early morning, we did not go to school that day, which was also great. We woke up that day, and Grandma told us that Dad had called earlier to tell us that the baby was born.

I was so excited. I couldn't wait to go home and meet the baby. The housekeeper was there when our grandparents took us home later that day. I gathered my siblings so we could help to clean the house for their arrival. We also made welcome home cards for Mommy and the baby. We were excited as we waited for them to come home.

But Dad came home alone late that evening. I remember how sad he looked when he told us the baby was very sick and needed to stay in the hospital. He said Mom was also not coming home as the doctors kept her for further observation. I was frightened and didn't understand what was happening. But even as a young child, I reassured myself that it didn't matter as long as my baby brother was alive. It didn't matter how long it took for him to come home. I was willing to wait to welcome him home. That night, I remember feeling very upset and confused and cried myself to sleep.

Nathan remained in the hospital for an extended period. When Mom returned home the following day, she explained that he required surgery and was in the intensive care unit for babies (NICU), making it impossible for us to visit him there. This news left me feeling deeply saddened and depressed.

A Big Sister's Heart

Finally, Mom informed us that we could meet him at the hospital. It was a quiet Sunday afternoon when Dad drove us there. We sat silently during the car ride, as Dad was never much of a talker. Nathan was still in the NICU, and we couldn't go in. So, the nurse carried him out to meet us at the entrance to the unit. He was almost a month old then but so tiny and frail. His eyes were closed, and he had a lot of tubes coming out of his body. The nurse was holding a small panda bear oxygen mask over his nose and mouth, and she had the tank in her other hand.

I was overwhelmed. I was momentarily lost, struggling to grasp the significance of what was happening to him. But then, as I told myself that none of that mattered, what mattered was that I got to see him. The nurse said we could touch his feet or legs. I kissed the soles of his feet and told him how happy I was to meet him finally and that we loved him and couldn't wait for him to come home. A penetrating sense of joy washed over me as I looked at him. Finally, I met my new brother! I was also taken aback by how fiercely protective I felt for him. He was so tiny. I knew then that I would do anything for him.

Our hospital visit was brief that day, and my heart ached when we had to leave. The days waiting for Nathan to return home were agonizing because I didn't just lose out on experiencing my brother's early days; I also felt like I lost Mom. She was hardly ever home since she left for the hospital each day before we headed to school and only returned at bedtime. Not having her around was tough, and I grew up a lot as I felt the need to shoulder more responsibilities. This included looking after my younger siblings, comforting them when they were scared, doing my best to answer their questions about what was happening, and assisting with household chores. I had less time for the things I wanted to do. But I didn't mind at all. I found comfort in knowing my brother wasn't alone at the hospital.

We also lost precious quality time with Dad, including our cherished bedtime ritual. It was a tradition he had upheld since we were little, where he would weave a continuous story featuring Sly Mongoose and Edward Bedward, characters from old Jamaican folklore. This storytelling journey spanned years, evolving as we grew older. Dad introduced new characters like the three Doberman dogs, two bulldogs, and a quirky poodle named

Crazzy. He even allowed us to contribute to the narrative as he spun it.

He concluded the bedtime story each night with the familiar Sly Mongoose song, "Sly Mongoose, your name gone abroad," and a promise of "next time on Sly Mongoose..."

The night before Nathan was born was the last time of this cherished tradition, as all our lives were forever changed.

When Nathan finally came home from the hospital, I felt like my prayers had been answered. I couldn't bear the thought of being separated from him again, so I was determined to assist in any way I could. Mom patiently showed me and my siblings how to hold him. I can still vividly recall the first time I cradled him; I was worried about hurting him because of the large bandage around his belly, and he was still tiny. But Mom arranged pillows around us to provide support.

As time passed, I eagerly helped with activities such as bathing him, placing him in his chair, assisting with feeding, and reading to him. As he grew older, these tasks became my duties, and I never stopped doing them. I also remember how Nathan often monopolized the TV, insisting on watching only the shows he liked. During dinner, he tended to pull down the tablecloth, sending everything crashing to the floor, and there were occasions when he would vomit or knock the food off the spoon to the floor. Cleaning up after him was quite a challenging task.

My Coping Mechanisms

Now that I am an adult, people often ask me, "What has your experience been like living with Nathan and his CP?" They asked apologetically, as if this was the worst thing that could have happened to my family. But the truth is, despite the added busyness, life with Nathan feels like a normal life to me because I've never known it any other way.

I learned early on to take everything in stride, and now, as a young adult, I'm committed to continuing to help. I stopped worrying about how much work it entailed because I realized that it was essential for Nathan's well-being, and I just want him to be happy. When I reflect on how I feel when I'm hungry, thirsty, or need a shower, I don't want Nathan to experience those discomforts.

My mom often refers to me as a "little mother" to Nathan, and she's probably right. With Nathan, my maternal instincts kicked in well before their time. Even when I'm away from home, I'll call Mom to check if he's been fed, bathed, or simply to ensure he's okay. She frequently reminds me that she is "Mom," but I see caring for Nathan as my responsibility, and I gladly embrace it.

I used to cry a lot when I saw how underdeveloped his body was. It deeply troubled me that so few therapy programs were available to him in Jamaica. However, I am now grateful that we live in the United States and that he has access to resources that were once beyond our reach in Jamaica. Seeing his remarkable progress in his physical, emotional, and cognitive development since his arrival here fills my heart with joy.

I also note that he has become more self-aware and quite opinionated. For example, he swats me away when he is annoyed because I kiss him too often or try to put face cream on him. I don't mind because it shows me he is becoming his own person, and I love that. I want my little brother to be happy, and I would do anything to bring him joy.

I also love and appreciate my parents for all they do to create opportunities for Nathan, my siblings, and me. This appreciation hit home for me strongly when Nathan was hospitalized for an intestinal blockage in April 2023. It was by being at the hospital that I realized how hard it was on them when he was in the hospital after his birth. They had to take care of him, my siblings, and me. The situation broke my heart, and I was too young to understand or help.

The Blessings of Nathan

When people see Nathan and see me helping him, I feel like they don't necessarily see how my little brother has inspired me and blessed my life. He has taught me to look beyond "self" and see and really see him. When I was younger, and people did something that annoyed me, I would brand them as "horrible." Having Nathan in my life, I no longer pass judgment on people. I now look beyond their behavior and realize an underlying reason must exist.

Forgiving and letting go is easier now. I have developed more tolerance and patience. He has also taught me to be more loving, careful, compassionate, understanding, and helpful.

From a big sister's perspective, Nathan has brought countless blessings into our lives. I hold dear the memories of the incredible adventures we embarked on, all thanks to Nathan. One such memory was when we spent several months in the USA at Ronald McDonald House for Nathan's intervention therapies. At the time, we were still living in Jamaica, so having the opportunity while we were getting his treatment to visit Disney World, Universal Studios, and SeaWorld through the Compassionate Partners Program was a once-in-a-lifetime experience. It remains one of my all-time favorites.

In addition, we did many fun things as a family, like a movie night in our parents' bedroom, where a projector was used to show the movie on the bedroom wall. We also went on adventures, such as visiting many of the famous rivers of Jamaica, like Reach Falls, Reggae Falls, Somerset Falls, Dunns River, and YS Falls. I loved that it wasn't just about work, but we had these remarkable family bonding experiences. I believe it became possible because of Nathan's disability, which, in an unexpected twist, unlocked precious gifts from our own creativity and through organizations such as the Compassionate Partners Program and the American Airlines Miles for Kids Program.

Caring for my brother brought our family closer together. We learned to celebrate even the most minor achievements and deeply understand the value of teamwork in supporting his daily needs. Our home has always been filled with love, laughter, and gratitude for our shared moments.

Where I Stand Today

I can't help but appreciate the unexpected development I have undergone because of helping to raise my brother Nathan. These include the development of strong advocacy skills, which I learned from watching my mother when I go with her and my dad to his therapy or medical appointments or during my mom's workshops and talks. I see how my mother navigates these appointments, especially when the practitioner is not hearing her. These experiences have taught me the importance of speaking up for those who can't and fighting for what's right. That was why I chose to be one of Nathan's legal guardians.

The most significant lesson I've learned from being the oldest child and sibling of a child with a disability is the beauty of diversity and the uniqueness of each individual. My brother's disability hasn't defined him; it's showcased his incredible strength and ability to touch hearts and change lives. He's taught me that our differences make us special and that true beauty lies in embracing those differences.

From where I now sit, I can honestly say that being the big sister of a child with cerebral palsy has been both challenging and rewarding.

TAKEAWAY

Adrianne's candid share helped me understand that a child's disability impacts every family member, often in unique ways shaped by their position within the family. The key lesson here underscores the significance of empowering parents with the knowledge and resources to establish a nurturing environment where every child in the household, regardless of age, can openly express themselves and be truly heard and supported.

Thanks to Adrianne's perspective as a loving big sister, the second key insight I've gained is an awareness of how our other children were often unintentionally sidelined during Nathan's crises. I've also come to recognize God's incredible grace and mercy that sustained her and her siblings, as they could have easily sought comfort and attention elsewhere. Yet, God's grace and mercy held them safe until we could truly listen and attend to their needs. I am eternally grateful.

CHAPTER 24

RYAN AND JORDANNE'S ACCOUNTS

Adrianne's sharing really got me thinking, prompting me to research to increase my understanding of how a child's disability affects other siblings in the household. I wanted to improve my parenting knowledge and skills to support my older children better as they went through this journey with Nathan.

I noticed a significant gap in research right from the start. A limited body of published work exists that addresses the intricate dynamics among siblings within special needs families. It is acknowledged siblings in such families often confront a range of distinct challenges. These challenges encompass a spectrum of emotions, from love and compassion to frustration and, at times, even resentment. These emotions are intricately linked to their siblings' condition. However, this particular aspect remains relatively unexplored in academic literature despite these complexities.

I wished I had fully grasped the importance of this aspect at the outset of our journey. Adrianne's revelation undeniably motivated me to converse openly and honestly with Ryan and Jordanne. Here's what each of them shared in their respective birth order.

RYAN

The Early Days

I am the second-born and the older brother of Jordanne and Nathan. I was six years old when Nathan was born. I remember when Dad and Mom told us that we would have a little baby, I prayed for a boy. I was very happy when they told us we had a baby boy. I don't have many memories of the time leading up to Nathan's birth. I just remembered that he stayed in the hospital when he was born, and we couldn't see him for a while. This made me sad.

I can still remember seeing Nathan for the first time in the hospital. He had all of these tubes going in and out of him, and I was scared because I didn't know what was happening. Mom and Dad told me that Nathan was sick and had surgery. But I was six years old and didn't understand what that meant. Even after Mom again explained what was happening with my baby brother, I still didn't understand. I expected him to look "normal" like other babies I had seen.

When he came home, I didn't look at him differently than my siblings. I was happy that I finally had a brother, played with him, and spent time with him. I didn't think about the fact that he couldn't walk or talk as he got older. It wasn't until other children at school started teasing me and calling my brother names that I realized that others saw him as different.

A Big Brother's Heart

I was in grade three then and was embarrassed when the kids asked what was wrong with him or teased me about him. Initially, I didn't know what to say and would be quiet. But after a time, the embarrassment gave way to anger, and I got into fights. My parents didn't know about the teasing and fights because I didn't want them to worry.

The cycle of embarrassment, anger, and fighting continued for a long time throughout the years. There were times when I cried when I got home. When my mom asked, I didn't know how to explain what was happening. So, I would tell her something else was happening and cry some more.

Eventually, my parents were called in to see the principal because I got into a fight with another kid. My mother started working with us to help us understand how to respond to others when they teased him. It was hard because I felt fiercely protective of him and my siblings.

I have always loved my brother, and I always will. However, I have had various challenges and emotional struggles in dealing with my younger brother's physical disability and being nonverbal. This included feeling a heightened sense of responsibility for Nathan's well-being, safety, and care at school, church, and whenever we went out. Even when my parents and older sister, Adrianne, were there, I still felt my responsibility as the older son was to care for everyone. It was emotionally taxing at times.

I often felt frustration and powerlessness when I saw Nathan's physical limitations and challenges in getting the needed services and help. As his older brother, this was the sibling I prayed for, and I wished I could do more to help or improve his life and living situation.

Truthfully, helping with Nathan's daily (and night) care was a struggle. It cut into my personal time, leaving me with fewer opportunities for my interests, hobbies, or social activities. For example, sometimes, in the middle of a video game match or contest, I would be called away by my parents or sisters to help feed Nathan, change the TV channel, or put him to bed. I resented that for a long time because it didn't leave me a lot of free time to hang out with friends or just be.

My Coping Mechanisms

But, as time passed, I learned how to channel my frustration and anger into sports. I played football (soccer), track and field, and got into parkour. This helped me deal with my anger. I also understood my brother's disability and special needs better. I was proud of him and all that he had overcome. I am not even sure when his disability stopped bothering me.

I didn't focus on his disability when I played with him. He loved the physical things we did, like roughhousing. Sometimes, my mom tried to get me to stop, but Nathan would start to complain if I did. He liked the fact that I didn't treat him as fragile or broken.

I also got heavily into video games. As I told my mom, it helped me to channel my frustrations, disappointments, and anger. As long as I was playing, I stayed out of my head. She understood and allowed me the space to play.

Eventually, I got help in learning how to put things into perspective. I learned to overcome my anger and frustration as I realized that my embarrassment was not about my brother's disability but about being teased.

Seeing my brother in the hospital this past April (2023) was very hard. I am a committed video game player, so I don't spend much time with him these days. But seeing him lying so small and helpless in the hospital bed made me regret that. I spent time with him then and vowed to always make time for him.

I have outgrown many of these struggles over the years. I also learned about his disability and now better understand how to support him and deal with some of these issues whenever they come up. I worry that as my life takes me to new places, I may no longer be at home to help with Nathan's care. I fear he will miss me and may not see me as often as he would like. I worry that as my parents age, some physical things they now do will become more difficult for them, and I may not be there to help them.

The Blessings of Nathan

On the other hand, Nathan has also helped me. He helped me appreciate that love has no barriers and no borders. He taught me to see God's creations as they are, not as I want them to be. He helped me see value and purpose in everything.

Just this past September (2023), I talked with Dad and Mom, thanking them for raising me in a Christian household and instilling Christian principles in my life. While I may not have always fully appreciated our time attending church, participating in private family devotions, reading the Bible, and praying together, growing older has given me a new perspective. I now understand that this foundational upbringing has significantly shaped my responses to life and how I navigate its challenges.

I firmly believe that with God, "every little thing will be all right." Yes, I pray for Nathan to get the support he needs to help him develop to his full potential and have a better quality of life. Here we are, living in the United States, where he has a much better quality of life.

Where I Stand Today

I do worry about the load of care on my parents now that my career has taken me away from home. They have done so much and sacrificed so much for me and my siblings. I want them to enjoy a better quality of life.

But most of all, I pray that God will continue to have His way in all our lives. I thank Him for His plans for Nathan, our family, and this world. Knowing that God, the Father of creation, has a plan for all of us assures me that all is well no matter what we face.

JORDANNE

The Early Years

I am the third child in our family, and for four years, I enjoyed the role of being the youngest before Nathan came along. I was still young and don't remember much about his early life. But I remember he didn't come home from the hospital immediately.

I have vivid memories of going with my dad, along with my brother and sister, to visit Nathan in the hospital. At that time, he was incredibly tiny, wrapped in bandages, and connected to various tubes, which was quite scary for me. The nurse brought him to us and said we could kiss his feet if we wanted to touch him. But I was hesitant and fearful, given his fragile condition. I worried that I might accidentally hurt him.

I distinctly recall my brother Ryan's refusal, saying, "I don't kiss people's feet." Despite my concerns, I kissed his feet, as I was also filled with happiness that I was meeting him.

My parents explained that Nathan was different, but at my young age, I didn't understand what that meant. I had no concept of a disability or how it affected someone. To me, he was simply my baby brother who needed extra care. When I looked at him, I wanted to protect and help him.

I still remember the first time I got to hold him. Mom positioned me on the living room couch, surrounded me with pillows, and carefully placed Nathan in my arms, showing me how to support his head and body properly. I felt an overwhelming sense of pride in that moment because it made me feel like a responsible grown-up actively contributing to my little brother's care. Looking back, I believe that was the beginning of the special bond that formed between us.

A Sister's Heart

I was always fiercely protective of Nathan. I distinctly remember the first time I assisted in changing his diaper. Mom had stepped outside to chat with a neighbor, and it happened that Nathan had a bowel movement. Adrianne, Ryan, and I decided to take the initiative and change him ourselves. Although it proved to be a bit challenging, we had observed Mom doing it so many times that we felt confident we could manage it.

At the time, I was around five years old, and my task was to pull the soiled diaper out from underneath him while Adrianne and Ryan lifted his legs. Unfortunately, I wasn't aware of the need to fold the diaper properly, so I flung it away, causing its contents to spill onto the rug and floor. Despite the mess, we were quite proud of our effort, and when Mom returned inside, we performed a little "ta-da" routine. Of course, she was both surprised that we had done it on our own and proud of our determination.

As the years passed, we all became experts at changing Nathan's diaper without any further mishaps.

When I was around eight years old, I was responsible for assisting Nathan with his homework. However, I faced a significant challenge because Nathan was nonverbal, and I wasn't sure how to help him effectively. I could sense that he knew the answers, but I struggled to find a way to facilitate his expression.

In my determination to help, I improvised and unknowingly created a communication board to aid him in expressing what he knew. Little did I realize at the time that this experience would serve as my initial introduction to the field of speech pathology, which I would later choose as my career path.

For a period, Nathan attended the same preparatory (elementary) school as Adrianne, Ryan, and me, and I looked out for him to make sure he was okay. I would secretly visit his classroom during the school day, and I loved how excited he got when he saw me. My protective instincts kicked in, and I made it a point to prevent any bullying or teasing directed at him.

I recall a time when Nathan was learning to isolate his fingers to pick things up, and he developed the habit of pinching. In an attempt to make him understand the discomfort it caused, there were moments when I pinched him back. Although it was done with good intentions, I always felt remorseful afterward. Thankfully, Nathan never held any grudges, and our bond remained strong.

My Coping Mechanism

While having Nathan as a brother has been a true blessing, I must admit that being a sibling to someone with special needs presented its fair share of challenges. It demanded a great deal of my free time and patience, particularly when it came to tasks like feeding him or assisting with his homework. It often felt like Nathan received special treatment due to his special needs, which sometimes meant that he seemed to get away with things like pinching us or monopolizing the TV, and it seemed like he always got his way.

It wasn't always fun and games for me. There were times when I felt somewhat invisible within our family dynamic. It seemed like there was always a crisis, whether it involved Nathan. Plus, Adrianne and Ryan frequently got into trouble at home. Because I was generally well-behaved and performed well in school, it sometimes felt like I didn't receive as much attention as the others.

Even though I was young, I also quickly recognized that my parents had their hands full, so I rarely shared my problems and often tried to figure things out independently. It's only recently that I opened up about these feelings with my mom, and to my surprise, she expressed her regret and apologized for not realizing the extent to which I had been handling things on my own instead of turning to her for support.

Setting high standards in my schoolwork was another coping strategy for me. I did not want to cause my parents to worry about me in this regard, so I became driven. Consequently, I placed considerable pressure on myself to excel academically.

Dancing was a primary coping strategy. My mom had enrolled me in ballet class when I was in the fourth grade, and I instantly fell in love with it. Dancing became my passion, something that was uniquely mine, and I cherished every performance. I remained dedicated to ballet throughout high school, eventually expanding my horizons to include cheerleading and exploring various dance forms, including reggae and hip hop. When I was dancing, I felt like I could truly be myself.

I still recall an embarrassing incident from one summer at Vocational Bible School (VBS). I was about six years old and found myself responsible for staying with Nathan for extended periods. Because Sunday school or children's Bible school couldn't accommodate him by himself, whenever Mom was teaching, it fell upon me to look after him, even if it meant taking him outside. On that particular day, Nathan had a meltdown as I wheeled his stroller back into the church hall because he didn't want to go back inside. It felt like everyone in the church auditorium turned to look at me. I was engulfed by a wave of emotions, including embarrassment, as I struggled to soothe him so that he would stop crying.

I also felt guilty for being embarrassed by anything about Nathan and his disability. Even then, I knew that being a special needs sibling involved a whirlwind of complicated feelings. However, I hadn't yet acquired the skills to effectively process these emotions, as I was still just a young child.

The Blessings of Nathan

Reflecting on those times from my current perspective, I can truly say that though the responsibilities were significant and sometimes overwhelming, I can appreciate the experience they brought into my life. This journey had a pivotal role in shaping my personal growth and development, instilling a strong sense of responsibility, commitment, and industriousness from a very young age. It taught me to navigate the delicate balance between my academic pursuits and my role in our home. I was part of something that was bigger than myself.

My mom often refers to my role with Nathan as a guiding light, leading me to my calling as a speech-language pathologist. It planted the seeds of compassion in my heart for helping special needs kids. I also remember the fun times we had traveling with Nathan to the USA for treatment when we lived in Jamaica. It opened the door for memorable experiences like visiting the Natural Science Center in Florida.

My parents went to great lengths to create enjoyable experiences and lasting memories for our family, and I will forever hold dear the moments we shared together. We had a family motto: "We all swim or sink, but none gets left behind." We truly lived by this mantra, and whether Mom was conducting workshops for teachers or parents, we were always actively involved.

I fondly remember those workshops, particularly the small soft mints she would place on the workshop tables. I relished the opportunity to assist with packing up afterward, mainly because it meant I could indulge in those mints to my heart's content.

As I share with my family, I do worry about Nathan's future, though not from the perspective of his care. I know my family, and we will always put measures in place to ensure he is well cared for. My worry is that he will see all of us—his siblings—grow up and move out on our own, have careers, get married, and have children. And he won't be able to experience any of that. I want Nathan to experience everything his heart desires, so it is difficult not knowing what the future holds in this aspect of his life.

Where I Stand Today

Nathan is a vital part of my life; we often agree that next to God, he is the family's anchor. We all love him unconditionally and will do everything to ensure he is happy and has all his needs met. I hope that we can increase his independence in the future, as I know this is something he would greatly appreciate.

Nathan stands as one of my greatest inspirations. I admire his strength and courage. I am so proud of him, my baby brother who overcame so much in his young life. His journey profoundly affects countless other children like him, who often remain invisible or excluded in our society.

TAKEAWAY

As I've often shared with others, I believe that God hand-picked each member of my family for the path we are walking. I am certain that Nathan's and our family's story would have taken a different course were it not for each of these children's unwavering support, boundless love, willingness to help, and deep commitment to Nathan and our family.

Furthermore, I feel incredibly blessed, deeply honored, and humbled for the privilege of being the mother of these extraordinary human beings. The lessons from these young children have shown that true compassion and empathy extend beyond our comfort zones, emphasizing the importance of meeting the needs of those we support. Their ability to forge a deep connection with their brother while nurturing mindfulness and kindness toward others fills my heart with gratitude.

Their stories have revealed that having a sibling with special needs can significantly shape character, fostering qualities like empathy, patience, responsibility, adaptability, and advocacy. This experience has instilled in them a deep bond, tolerance, and resilience, making them compassionate advocates who champion the rights and acceptance of individuals with disabilities in society.

CHAPTER 25

NATHAN'S ACCOUNT: THIS GIFT FROM GOD

Beneath the Surface

It is of utmost importance to provide the context for this chapter, as it serves as a compelling testimony to Nathan's true identity as intended by God and the acknowledgment of the precious gift he embodies. As I shared in the preceding chapters, I was divinely assured that this child was a gift from God, setting my mind on a natural course and shaping my expectations for what this truly meant.

In the early days of my pregnancy, when I thought about the term "gift," I only knew how it was usually used. The definitions in dictionaries encompass concepts such as "a notable capacity, talent, or endowment."[33] Another set of definitions includes "something given to someone, often on a special day" and un-

---

33 "Gift," Merriam-Webster, accessed November 15, 2023, **https://www.merriam-webster.com/dictionary/gift**.

derscores the connection to a "natural ability or talent."[34] One of my favorite definitions characterizes a gift as "something that is bestowed or acquired without any particular effort."[35]

As you can imagine, I was elated that my unborn child was undeniably unique, even though I was not yet sure in what ways. Upon receiving his diagnosis, I struggled to interpret it within the context of a "gift." However, as I reached that turning point and embraced our path, I recognized the need for divine guidance to see beyond the physical appearance and truly perceive.

Learning to see my son through God's eyes was a journey that involved prayer, deep listening, self-reflection, and the unwavering support of my tribe, comprising both family and professionals. In this process, I came to realize that my initial expectations were creating barriers. My mind had painted vivid pictures of him excelling in academics and the arts or standing out in some extraordinary way. I even let my imagination wander, envisioning him as a sports sensation akin to legendary countrymen like Usain Bolt, Asafa Powell, and Yohan Blake—encounters with these icons that remain vivid in my memory. I also entertained thoughts of him possessing musical talents, much like the iconic Bob Marley or Jimmy Cliff, or perhaps becoming a brilliant academic star or a source of inspiring spiritual leadership.

Letting go of my preconceived expectations was the first crucial step in seeing the real Nathan beneath the surface. This process required time, unwavering perseverance, and a good deal of patience. But once I managed to release those expectations, my eyes of understanding were truly opened, allowing me to see my

---

34 "Gift," Cambridge Dictionary, accessed November 15, 2023, **https://dictionary.cambridge. org/us/dictionary/english/gift.**
35 "Gift," Collins Online Dictionary, accessed November 15, 2023, **https://www.collinsdictionary.com/us/dictionary/english/gift.**

son for who he is.

I remember praying often, saying, "Lord God, please help me to see Nathan through Your eyes." Remarkably, God answered my prayers by bringing people like my friends Dawn, Senta, and Erin into my life, gradually shifting my perspective. He also introduced me to some remarkable individuals with disabilities, some of whom I will talk about in the upcoming chapters. These encounters offered me fresh perspectives that allowed me to appreciate and understand the remarkable child that Nathan is truly.

What Nathan is about to share has been thoughtfully gathered from numerous conversations I've had over the years, where I've shared about him or introduced him to educators, clinicians, and specialists. These discussions have consistently emphasized his identity beyond his disability.

Additionally, in June 2023, Nathan's special education and transition team at school took a significant step by creating a person-centered plan for him. This collaborative effort involved various aspects of his life, bringing together teachers, paraprofessionals, nurses, guidance counselors, case managers, and family members to gain a comprehensive understanding of Nathan's likes, dislikes, aspirations, and strengths. This approach was essential because Nathan has developed various communication methods tailored to specific groups he interacts with.

I chose to write Nathan's perspective in the first person as a means to raise awareness and promote understanding of the crucial importance of giving a voice to those who may not have one. This was done with the utmost care, empathy, and respect for his unique experiences and preferences.

NATHAN

As a nonverbal child with cerebral palsy, I am the youngest of four children for my parents, Robert and Christine. My family loves me, and I love them dearly. I know that they are all fully committed to supporting me in leading a happy and independent life.

My life has been quite challenging. I was born with a birth defect, underwent surgery at just three days old, spent twenty-four days in the hospital, and received a diagnosis of cerebral palsy when I was only nine months old. My family has always taken great care of me, but I know they are also worried about what my life will be like as I grow older.

I'm used to being the baby of my family. My parents often say I'm the boss of everybody, and I absolutely love it. My family is a fun and lively bunch; we laugh and play a lot. I love it most when we do goofy things together, like dancing around while watching my favorite movies or cartoons. They even act out scenes with me, which cracks me up every time. I love musicals, especially Disney's *Frozen*, *Encanto*, *Hercules*, *The Lion King*, and *The Little Mermaid*, especially the live-action version of the last one. I burst into laughter every time my mom, dad, and sisters put towels on their heads and pretend to be Elsa's cape and hair so they can throw them off at the end of the song, "Let it Go." I also love it when we do things together as a family, like going to Church, the movies, or to the park.

I know the world does not see me like my family does. When they first meet me, many people judge my abilities based on my physical presentation. After all, I fill up any space I am in with my big wheelchair and someone pushing it to get me around;

people always notice me when I enter a room.

I often notice people's reactions when they see me. Some seem embarrassed, others quickly avert their eyes, and a few look right through me. My mom has explained that these reactions occur because many people haven't learned how to engage with people who, like me, are different. She also said some people may not understand my disability and its impact on me, including how I communicate using a device. It sometimes brings me down when they ignore me, even when I speak to them, or they speak over me as if I'm invisible.

I want people to understand that I'm much more than just my cerebral palsy. My disability is only one aspect of who I am. Just like everyone else, I am created in the image and likeness of God. Admittedly, my disability presents challenges in everyday tasks like walking, talking, feeding myself, or being fully independent. However, I am right here, present and eager to engage with the world. I hope that people can see me for who I am, interact with me, and offer me the same opportunities to engage with them in return.

Label Jars, Not People

All too often, when people see me, they are quick to attach labels like "afflicted," "helpless," "disabled," "handicapped," "wheelchair-bound," "burden," "pitiable," "incapable," or "unproductive." But they are not so quick to understand the harm in labeling people, especially those like me with disabilities. When I was much younger, I used to overhear people in my school community arguing in my presence, and they would often claim that I couldn't understand what they were saying or ask questions like why my parents were wasting money to send me to school since I couldn't learn. My caregiver, Danielle, would frequently speak up for me, insisting that I understood what they were saying. Sadly, they often didn't believe her.

I often find myself in adult company because I require assistance with everyday life functions. Sometimes, they engage in inappropriate conversations, forgetting that I am there or assuming that I don't understand. I want them to be mindful that I'm listening and understanding what they're saying.

It is important to me that people know that I am fearfully and wonderfully made. My voice may be different, but my thoughts and understanding are as real as anyone else's. I want everyone to know that I am none of those labels.

Another misconception that I often encounter is that some people see me as a burden because I rely on others for assistance. They often say things to my family or caregiver like, "I don't know how you manage taking care of him," or "I couldn't do what you are doing," or "You are strong to be taking care of him every day." I want to remind them that everyone needs help at some point in their lives, and I'm no exception to that. When I receive the right support and services, such as occupational and physical therapy, and when I'm encouraged to use aids like my communication device, I can learn how to do some things for myself. Like everyone else, I desire to be as independent as possible.

Another frustrating experience I often face is when I visit new specialists, therapists, or service providers, and they ignore me, talking only to my parents about me as if I am not there. They discuss helping me but often don't take the time to communicate with me directly or wait for my feedback. I love meeting new people and being included in conversations about me. I'm also learning to use my communication device to express myself, my feelings, and my needs. All I ask is for the space and opportunity to do so. I always carry my device with me; please use it to communicate with me. It helps me to build my voice. When you don't use it, it takes away my voice.

My guidance counselor class taught me that my voice and feelings matter. I want to be included in the decision-making process concerning me. Give me the opportunities to exercise my right to be actively involved in my own life and have a say in the choices that affect me.

My Strengths

Just like everyone else, I have distinctive qualities that make me uniquely me. One of the things that sets me apart is my distinctive smile, which I'm quite well known for.

My smile. My mom often refers to my smile as my million-dollar gift to the world because it has a way of touching people's hearts. She tells me it was one of the very first skills I mastered, even when I was just a baby. She recalls how, back then, a physical therapist in Jamaica noticed my smile and predicted that it would open doors for me in the world. The therapist says my smile draws people into my joy and warmth. She also mentioned that I have a "mellow" personality, which naturally attracts people to me. This is great because I love people and love to share my smile with them.

Smiling at people and witnessing their smiles in return has always filled me with immense joy. I often laugh heartily when they do; it becomes a joyfully blessed exchange. Whenever I encounter someone who appears sad or stressed, I offer them a smile to brighten their day.

At school, I am frequently told that my smile has the ability to brighten everyone's day, and that warms my heart. It makes me feel like I'm positively impacting someone else's life. This is how I connect with the world around me, and it brings me immeasurable joy.

My love for God. My parents have always told me that children with special needs, like me, are close to God's heart and that He watches over us to protect us. I believe them wholeheartedly because I have a deep and unexplainable love for the Lord God. Going to church with my family is one of my favorite things to do. Even though it has been challenging, as many churches cannot accommodate my needs—no ramps for my wheelchair, no accessible bathrooms, and no inclusive Sunday school or church programs—I still love going because it is the house of God.

One of my favorite moments at church is singing praise and worship songs. I get caught up in the music and feel incredibly close to God, especially when we all join together, raising our hands in praise. It's a moment of pure connection and spirituality that fills my heart with joy. I also have a deep love for the reading of the Bible and the preaching.

I always stay with my parents during the church service, and while I sometimes wish I could attend Sunday school like other kids my age, I don't mind because I get to be in God's presence, no matter where I sit. After the service ends, I like to remain in my seat until the choir finishes singing, just soaking in the beauty of it all.

Leading up to my health episode in April 2023, I was drawn

to watching the livestream services from our church back in Jamaica all day. It felt like God was reassuring me that He was with me no matter what I went through. This support sustained me during my surgery and hospitalization, which was exceptionally challenging.

I continue to spend time with God through the live stream services daily. I have a deep faith that Jesus loves me just as I am. I greatly love Him for everything He does for me, my family, and people around me worldwide.

Loving-kindness. Being kind and loving toward each other holds great importance in my life. In my family, they lovingly refer to me as our home's "hug-o-meter." For example, when a family member is about to leave, it's become a tradition for me to ensure that they hug everyone before departing. If someone is missed, I make sure to call their attention to it. I give my thumbs-up of approval once they have hugged everyone. Even if we have visitors, I also make sure they get a hug.

Human connection. I love connecting with people. I'm friendly and openly welcome people regardless of their background. I know that this sometimes embarrasses my family when I warmly greet complete strangers when we're out and about. Sometimes, these strangers respond, and other times, they don't. But none of that really matters to me. What's important to me is that they know I see them, and I want them to feel acknowledged and appreciated for who they are.

I remember one time I was at the dentist's office with my mom and dad. Another teenager like me, who has CP and is nonverbal, came in with his family, and as I passed by, I couldn't resist but smile, wave, and say "ello," which is how I greet people. His family waved back, to my delight, and I got even more excited, continuing to wave at them.

Later, when we were leaving, my mom stood with me, waiting for Dad to bring the minivan to pick us up. The family and the kid from the dentist's office happened to pass by, and the mom asked my mom if I was a friend of their son from school or therapy. They were surprised to learn that we lived in a different township, quite far from them, and I didn't go to the same school as their son or share any common circles.

My mom explained that I love to connect with new people, especially when they are like me. The family responded by saying they loved that about me. That day, I made some new friends, making me happy as we drove away.

I must have gotten that from my mom, who often strikes up conversations with complete strangers when we're out and about, and she doesn't even need to know their names. She's just as warm and friendly as I am, and I love our ability to connect with people and create positive moments.

Discerning spirit. My family often describes me as having a strong sense of discernment. They first discovered this when I was much younger, and my mom was conducting job interviews to select my caregiver. During one particular interview, she had to leave the room briefly and asked the lady to hold me. However, to everyone's surprise, I refused to go to the lady, which my mom found quite telling.

As a result, my mom decided to include me in the remaining interviews. She noticed that I displayed hesitation toward some people and was more willing to approach others. However, when I met Danielle, something clicked within me. Even though I was just two years old then, my mom humorously referred to it as my "warmth meter." I immediately went to Danielle and hugged her, and that's how she became my caregiver, one of my best friends, and an extended family member for more than ten years.

This unique ability of mine to discern continued to be valuable. When my grandparents were hiring a caregiver for my grandmother, my mom included me in the interview process despite my age four. Mom recalls that there was one lady I didn't even want to touch me, and later, background checks revealed that she had a history of dishonesty, mean-spiritedness, and stealing from her past employers. The person I helped them choose became an extended member of our family, just like Danielle, and cared for me as I grew older.

Equally, I know when people mean me well and when they don't. I know when they pretend in front of my parents that they are good to me when they are not. I am glad my parents know this about me, which has helped them know when something is wrong at school throughout the years.

Sense of humor. I also have a mischievous streak of physical humor that can be downright contagious. If, by chance, you happen to stub your toe, take an unexpected tumble, or encounter any physical mishap in my presence, brace yourself for an uproarious fit of laughter. I don't know why, but I find these situations to be incredibly funny. Sometimes, I laugh so hard that I can hardly catch my breath. On occasion, I'll laugh for days whenever I see the person involved and remember what happened.

People who know me well can spot the mischievous twinkle in my eye when unexpected situations unfold, and they're well aware that my hearty laughter is about to burst forth. Through these moments, I've learned my sense of humor can shatter barriers and disappear any preconceived notions others might hold about me. It's an enduring reminder that my disability doesn't shape my identity; rather, it's just one thread in the vibrant fabric of my life.

Determined. My mom often describes me as having stubborn determination. She says this determination helped me survive in her womb and overcome the challenges of my birth, childhood, and surgery. She calls it my "will to live." But as she and those who know me have discovered, I carry this determination with me in everything I do. So, when I come across a therapy exercise I don't particularly enjoy, when I get bored with my schoolwork, or when I simply don't want to transition from what I'm doing, that same willpower can sometimes transform into a stubborn and determined refusal to cooperate.

Often, this behavior communicates that I'm feeling bored, tired, or uncomfortable with what I'm doing; you will notice that I might display signs of frustration on my face, use body language like slouching or avoiding eye contact, resist by pulling away or pushing objects, make vocalizations of displeasure, become restless or fidgety, engage in repetitive behaviors, or simply refuse to participate.

On my communication devices, I am learning to select symbols or words indicating my feelings, and it's important for my caregiver, teachers, and therapists to interpret these nonverbal cues and adapt activities or therapy exercises to create a supportive and responsive environment that respects my emotions and preferences.

Justice and inclusion. As someone living with a lifelong

disability, I intimately understand these concepts beyond mere words. I experience them every single day when systems and people often overlook me and people like me when developing programs and services. I've been a paying student in classrooms where I am still excluded. Once, I was the only student with a disability and the only one who was never put into any sports day activities. I watch my mom tirelessly advocate for me and see how many administrators are unaware of my need and right to be included.

As I got older, I noticed the invitations to birthday parties stopped coming. People don't seem to understand that I am, first and foremost, a person who wants inclusion and friendship. I want to be part of the group, to have friends who share the joys of childhood with me. This situation sometimes makes me feel like I don't belong anywhere apart from home.

So, because I understand what it is like to be left out, I point it out to the adult in the room when someone is left out. I use eye gaze, pointing, and sounds to draw attention to those who are being overlooked.

My family says I have a remarkable talent for remembering people and their faces. From my vantage point in my wheelchair, I often spot people before my family does, and I never hesitate to call out to them. My mom loves to share a heartwarming story about her friend, Aunty Andria. I was out with Dad at the local supermarket in Jamaica one day when I saw Aunty Andria in the distance. She didn't see us, so I called out to her with un-containable excitement until she noticed me. Aunty Andria was taken aback by how excited I was to see her and by how eagerly I opened my arms for a hug. Even after all these years, Aunty Andria still tells the story of how I made her day and made her feel special.

At the end of the day, I want people to understand that beneath my disability lies a person who, just like them, wants to belong, have friendships, be included, and be given the support and opportunities to participate fully in all aspects of life.

TAKEAWAY

Unlocking Nathan's voice was a journey that took years, spanning his entire life. However, when I finally succeeded, I discovered an interesting person with a wealth of thoughts and a fascinating personality. One common pitfall that able-bodied individuals often make is assuming that because we work with a particular population, we know all individuals with similar disabilities. However, I've learned the importance of maintaining an inclusive posture involving Nathan in decisions regarding our household and himself.

In addition, Nathan's distinctive perspective and life experiences have truly been my most profound teachers, refining my capacity to discern the divine presence in each and every person. In his own unique manner, Nathan has illuminated a profound truth: God's love knows no bounds. Regardless of our abilities or disabilities, Nathan has shown me that every individual is born with a unique purpose, a divine calling that rises above earthly distinctions. It's a lesson steeped in love, embracing inclusivity, and celebrating the boundless grace of God.

CHAPTER 26

FINDING HARMONY WITH GOD'S MASTER PLAN

In the chapters you've journeyed through, I've shared the stories, pivotal moments, people, and defining experiences that shaped our incredible journey in raising Nathan. When we began, I confess, I couldn't see any silver lining to our situation. In those early years, questions filled my mind about his disability and the uncertain path ahead: *Where was the promised gift from God? How could I best support and guide this unique child? What would the future hold for him, and what purpose or lesson did this journey hold? How would I cope with everything?*

Although I had been a Christian long before Nathan was born, his arrival and subsequent diagnosis offered me a new beginning—to discover who God is on a deeper level and to uncover my own identity in Him more purposefully. Raising Nathan became a journey of shedding my old mindset and the doubts and

uncertainties that came with it, propelling me onto a transformative path that aligned with God's master plan for me, Nathan, my
family, and my work. What had initially been a landscape dominated by fear, anxiety, and confusion gradually unveiled itself as
a sacred journey adorned with blessings and extraordinary gifts.

In his unique and beautiful way, Nathan brought these gifts
into our lives and generously shared them with the wider world.
I have since learned that our voyage was much more than overcoming challenges; it was about the journey of self-discovery,
family, love, resilience, faith, and purpose. On a spiritual level,
I came to understand that God places more importance on the
journey than the destination, conveying the notion that there is
purpose in every process. On a practical note, the path of raising
a child with disabilities is multifaceted, demanding dedication,
resilience, and a supportive network. It entails addressing practical challenges while also nurturing the child's holistic development, well-being, and potential and taking care of oneself.

This is why, in God's design, we aren't meant to undertake
it alone. In fact, going alone is impossible without it affecting
both the child and the parent(s)' physical, mental, and psychological well-being.[36] Therefore, God strategically brings people into
our lives to assist us on this journey. Though I now recognize
this in hindsight, God strategically brought people and resources
into my life at different points, each contributing a vital building block that helped create the pathway to His plan for us. One
particularly influential story in my journey is that of Brigette and
her son, Adam.

My first connection with them happened many years before

36 Dennis J. Baumgardner, "Social Isolation Among Families Caring for Children With Disabilities," Journal of patient-centered research and reviews 6, no. 4 (2019):229-232, **https://doi.
org/10.17294/2330-0698.1726.**

I became a parent. It came through a colleague at work who, as it turned out, was Brigette's sister-in-law. She talked about them frequently, and her admiration for them ran deep. She would often recount Brigette's unflinching passion and proactive advocacy for her son Adam's rights as a child with a disability.

In 2007, almost a decade later, Brigette resurfaced in my thoughts with remarkable force as I organized my first special education workshop. She stood out as the only parent I knew who had initiated a social movement to give voice to her son's educational barriers. I believed her presence and story would add depth to the workshop.

Not knowing exactly what to anticipate, I was completely enthralled by her words as she spoke, for they sowed the seeds of hope deep within my spirit. Only through reflection, as I sat by Nathan's side, I recognized the parallels and realized that Brigette's story had been an inspirational roadmap I had used to navigate my journey. It became clear how her shared wisdom played an instrumental role in helping me find harmony in God's plan. Recently, I reached out to Brigette to remind her of that story and ask permission to share it in this book. I am grateful that she graciously consented. She revisited the presentation she gave in 2007, providing an updated glimpse of how Adam is faring today as a young adult. Here is the account she presented back in 2007, which she has since updated to offer insights into Adam's current journey.

MY PLATE—IN PRIDE OF PLACE

The first emotion I felt was, *Surely, this couldn't be happening to me.* Then came anger, a resounding "Why me, dear God? Why would You do this to me?" And eventually, guilt crept in, whispering that I must have done something to deserve this, to cause this to my child. "What terrible sin had I committed that You should visit this on me, that You had to punish me and my child this way?" Then I went into grief because I kept thinking of the perfect baby that I did not have.

My son Adam was born twelve years ago with spina bifida.[37] He is paralyzed from the waist down. And then I got a gift—a plate—that I have on display in my home in pride of place.[38]

That plate was the most beautiful thing I had seen. The colors had subtle hues of turquoise and brown, and cobalt blue blended to form a pattern that was as intricate as it was simple—it was breathtaking.

And then it occurred to me that it didn't start out breathtaking. It started out as a lump of clay. Someone dug that clay out of the ground and delivered the lump of dirt to the artist. The artist then kneaded the dirt, like dough, until it changed and became malleable and shapeable, and when it was the right consistency, the artist had to mold it into the shape she envisioned that she saw in her mind's

---

37 Spina bifida is a congenital condition where the spinal cord, spinal column, or both do not fully develop due to the incomplete closure of the neural tube during fetal development. It can result in various spinal cord and nerve-related problems, with severity ranging from mild (spina bifida occulta) to severe (myelomeningocele).

38 "Giving something pride of place" in this context means to prominently display or position something in a way that highlights its importance or significance. It signifies that the item or object is given a position of honor or distinction, often in a prominent location or setting, to emphasize its value or sentimental meaning. This phrase is commonly used when talking about displaying cherished possessions, artwork, or objects of significance in a home or public space.

eye. And when it was formed, she placed it into a kiln and heated it up at four hundred degrees.

When it came out, the artist diligently applied the dull and lifeless glazes in the pattern she envisioned in her mind's eye. When she was done, she placed it back in the oven, cranked the temperature to five hundred degrees, and fired it again. What emerged, like a butterfly from a chrysalis, was my breathtakingly beautiful plate.

At that moment, I understood, and, like Saul, I had a revelation. We are exposed to our own kneading, molding, forming, and firing, and if we want to emerge from our chrysalis as beautiful objects, we need to embrace these processes. The kneading and molding are not there to break us but rather to form, fire, and allow our full colors to shine through. What is important is how we face our challenges and allow them to influence us.

In that moment, I realized that I needed to mourn the loss of that perfect child—the child who would walk, then run, and perhaps play cricket or football—so that I could be the best mother that I could be to the child I did have, who is perfect in his own way. I decided that if I was going to shake myself out of my depression, it had to be for something big. So, I created a big future for my child. I wanted him never to see himself as confined to a wheelchair, even though he used one, because the world would be his for the taking. I wanted him to never feel limited in terms of what he knew he could accomplish. And the role for me as his parent was to make it so!

At this moment, I realized that if I was going to create this reality for my child, I had to stop thinking about myself and stop wallowing in my grief. I had to start being unreasonable and intentional—I had to recognize what needed to be done and then do it. I started by first going back to school to study social policy research and advocacy for social change. I changed careers and started a support group for parents of children with disabilities. Every time I felt overwhelmed, I would renew my commitment to the vision I had created and press forward.

Learning to be a parent of a child with a disability was my challenge, but it was pivotal and essential to my and my family's survival, which resulted in my life passion. Many of us experience fear with things we really want to accomplish, and some of us experience fear of the unknown. In these instances, what we need to do is to be courageous, to acknowledge the fear, and to act anyway. The only way to get to that wonderful relationship with our sons or daughters, the perfect job, or the new business is to be courageous. Don't say "Poor me" and give in; instead, face the challenge, accept where you are starting—create a vision and a plan, and work toward it daily.

Adam has not let his challenge of using a wheelchair stop him from setting big goals and working toward them. He attended one of the leading high schools here in Jamaica and today is a university student pursuing his dream to become a human resource professional.

Brigette Levy

As I looked at Nathan peacefully sleeping in his hospital bed, I realized just how much I had learned from that time. Little did I know then that I was actually embodying all the key actions she had stressed: embracing the process, facing my fears and challenges head-on, following what I believed God was urging me to do even when it didn't completely make sense to me—envisioning a brighter future for Nathan, being deliberate in my actions, recognizing what needed to be done and taking action, making a career change, and pursuing graduate studies to contribute to research and innovation in the field of disabilities. The journey demanded even more courage than I could summon on my own, pushing me to rely heavily on God, the one constant, every step of the way.

At that moment, it became clear to me how this analogy powerfully mirrors the profound truth that God utilizes these life experiences to mold us into the unique and beautiful lives envisioned for each of us. Every journey, guided by divine intent, unfolds as a purposeful and distinctive masterpiece.

Nathan stirred, opened his eyes, and immediately looked at the NG tube snaking across his chest and bed, leading to the gastric drainage jar slowly filling up. His determined spirit was evident as his eyes widened in protest. He was clearly making progress, and he seemed eager to have the tubes removed. While I knew that this phase of his recovery would keep us on high alert, trying to prevent him from dislodging or pulling out the tubes, I felt a growing sense of hope and confidence that he would successfully recover from this health event.

CREATING A BIG FUTURE FOR NATHAN

The most challenging part of Brigette's advice was creating a vision and plan for Nathan. *How could I envision a brighter future when I had such a limited understanding of his disability and felt unsure about how to help him?* It took me a while to fully grasp this concept. It often felt like trying to play a game of chess without a clear understanding of the rules, and to make it even more complex, it was as if some crucial chess pieces were conspicuously absent from the board. Not long after that, I stumbled upon a book titled *Perspectives from the Jamaican MAP (Motto, Anthem, and Pledge)*, and I had the honor of meeting its author, Yvonne O. Coke, affectionately known as Ms. Yvonne. Both the book and extensive conversations with Ms. Yvonne were pivotal in deepening my understanding of my Jamaican identity and our sacred mission, as articulated in our national pledge, which commits us to "advancing the welfare of the whole human race."[39]

This was the point where I began piecing everything together, discerning the path I believed God was guiding me toward, which ultimately shaped my vision and plan for Nathan and myself. I started to view caregiving as an act of service to God. Although Nathan is my son, I recognize that he is, first and foremost, God's precious child. How I cared for him held deep significance to God, echoing the scripture, "Whatever you did for one of the least of these brothers and sisters of mine, you did for me."[40] This

---

39 "Anthem & Pledge," Jamaica Information Service, accessed November 15, 2023, **https://jis. gov.jm/information/anthem-pledge/**.
40 Matthew 25:40 (NIV)

perspective also framed my work with children with disabilities and their families.

During our conversations, Ms. Yvonne frequently emphasized a crucial point: that God has a purpose for bringing Nathan into this world, and his story is still unfolding. This perspective had a profound impact on my vision for both Nathan and me. I invited Ms. Yvonne to contribute her testimony of Nathan's journey to this book, and she graciously shared this beautiful reflection with me.

> I met Christine, Nathan's mother, through a mutual friend. As we spoke, we discovered that we had a shared love of God and a common vision for our beloved nation, Jamaica, albeit from different perspectives. As I shared with Christine from the first time we met, Nathan is undoubtedly a precious gift from God. He embodies so much of Jamaica's untapped potential.
>
> As I also shared in her first account of this book, her books on raising Nathan are God-commissioned, as Nathan is the perfect evangelist for the cause of people with disabilities. He is armed with real weapons of disarmament, chief of which his mother calls "His killer smile," which he has learned to skillfully unleash. When unleashed upon unsuspecting victims, Nathan's heart-warming smile arrests and renders them powerless to turn away without a positive response.
>
> Nathan's eyes have a unique quality that transcends human understanding and highlights the essential

need we all have for unconditional love. This compels us to lay aside every weight and is a gift of God to Jamaica in her quest to fulfill the nation's purpose. He is here to point us to and challenge Jamaica's nation to keep our pledge, "Before God and all mankind...to...play [our] part in advancing the welfare of the whole human race."[41]

Observing him reminds me of the essential quality of patience, which is the very first attribute of love. If we are to realize the vision outlined in our nation's MAP (motto, anthem, and pledge), we must pursue it with untiring patience, as patience is a hallmark of maturity, a quality that Nathan embodies so beautifully.

Spending time with Nathan often brings tears to my eyes, not out of pity for him, but because I grieve for those of us who fixated on his physical challenges and overlook the brilliant light he shines on our own spiritual and mental limitations. We sometimes fail to grasp that he not only carries a profound message but that he himself is the embodiment of that message, one meant for "the whole human race." In our failure to understand this, we miss the essence of his message.

How can someone who has faced such profound physical challenges exude such unbridled joy and happiness? What deep insights might Nathan possess, ones he has yet to share with us? What lies

41 "Anthem & Pledge," Jamaica Information Service, accessed November 15, 2023, **https://jis. gov.jm/information/anthem-pledge/**.

ahead on his remarkable journey? How can any of us question the worth of Nathan's life? These thoughts have crossed my mind as I've witnessed his personal growth over time. True to his name, Nathan is indeed a gift—a gift bestowed upon us all to prompt introspection about our own lives and the inherent value within each of us, regardless of outward appearances.

We do not get to choose God's purpose for creating humanity in His image and likeness; instead, we are granted the privilege of observing and learning from each life that crosses our path. Nathan's story is still unfolding, and he invites all of us to contribute to its narrative. The roles we play in shaping this story become a part of the Earth's history, revealing how each of us, when given the opportunity, can uncover and nurture the rarest forms of beauty—much like a diamond hidden deep within the Earth, waiting for the skilled hands to discover, mine, cleanse, and cut it to reveal its perfection.

Nathan's village, composed of those entrusted with his care, enjoys the extraordinary chance to unleash his inner beauty upon our world.

Yvonne O. Coke

True to his nature, Nathan's inner beauty radiated brilliantly during his hospital stay. I witnessed the sheer delight he brought to the entire hospital team. Every day, when I walked in, different individuals would express how his smile had brightened their day. Even nurses, regardless of whether they were assigned to him or not, would make a point of visiting the room just to bask in the warmth of his signature smile. The technicians and clinicians, whether they were there for radiology tests or therapy like chest therapy, physical therapy, and occupational therapy, couldn't help but be uplifted by his presence.

As Nathan's strength returned, my spirit soared despite the physical ways he communicated that he was ready to go home. His attempts to remove his NG tubes, complaints, and constant pointing to the room door signified he was done and wanted to leave. In a matter of days, this escalated to him making daring attempts to scale the bedrails in his resolute quest for freedom.

He was discharged a week later and cleared after another week to return to school and his activities. His school community welcomed him back with joy and celebration, and he celebrated his nineteenth birthday with his peers.

On Nathan's birthday, May 4, 2020, I sat in quiet reflection and gratitude. His life had already made a significant difference in the lives of so many people. He has proven to us that having a disability doesn't imply a lack of ability. Instead, he has inspired countless people to recognize that disability is a part of the human condition and can be a genuine, practical, and inspiring aspect of life. He motivates others to become more attentive, get involved, and actively participate in life. His story drew numerous specialists to Jamaica through the Nathan Ebanks Foundation, where thousands of teachers receive disability-specific training for the first time. Thousands of parents have received hands-on training, and hundreds of children have received their first (and often only) speech evaluations. Through this work, we have witnessed children with physical disabilities taking their first steps or learning to feed themselves. We have established a care model for supporting children with disabilities in children's homes that continues to benefit these children. Though we no longer live in Jamaica, Nathan's legacy has had a lasting impact on the inclusivity of Jamaica's landscape, policies, and practices.

Nathan possesses a remarkable talent for forming deep soul connections with others, demonstrating that even in the midst of challenges, we can unearth hope and joy. He also inspires those around him to reflect on their own limitations and actively embrace hope in their lives in spite of what they may be going through. It was intriguing to observe that the scars from his two surgeries had created a prominent cross-shaped imprint spanning from his chest to his abdomen. This enduring symbol serves as a constant reminder that we have come this far by faith and that God, who has started a good thing, will see it through to completion.

We experienced a profound full-circle moment on his high school graduation day. He received a resounding standing ovation as he was wheeled across the stage, radiating joy and animation, to proudly collect his diploma. He had met the graduation requirements despite all the formidable odds that had stood against him throughout the course of his young life.

Tears welled up, blinding me, as someone close to me reached out and said, "That is all for your son!" The auditorium echoed with cheers, applause, and jubilation. I was astonished that in just three short years of living in the United States and attending high school, he had managed to nurture such a close-knit community within a mainstream school where he was one of only a few children with disabilities.

Today, he is a "super senior" in high school, part of the 18-21 transition-to-adult-life program. He eagerly steps out each day to catch his bus and returns home brimming with excitement. As our past has taught me, each stage of his development brings forth new gifts, blessings, and opportunities, some of which may appear as challenges, along with new expressions of God. I can't wait to see what God unfolds in him and through him in this next chapter of his life.

TAKEAWAY

In Nathan's hospital room, I had my own eureka moment, realizing that God had used individuals like Brigette to plant seeds of hope in my heart. Much like her words, I had become "unreasonable," "intentional," "confronting challenges head-on." I had learned to accept and embrace the process as necessary to the unfolding of God's plan in our lives. Ms. Yvonne empowered me to take purposeful action and remain steadfast in the journey. Through her prayerful counsel, the steadfast support of my village community, which includes my home pastor, Rev. Dr. Merrick "Al" Miller, Tara Caroll Sanchez, my dear sister in Christ, a passionate professional collaborator from Texas, and numerous others who have chosen to join us on this journey, I have gained clarity regarding the vision for our lives. With the blessings of this amazing network, I was able to craft a personalized development plan for Nathan and his future, aligning it with God's master plan for us and through us, and watched God breathe life into it, even in the face of great odds.

I learned the importance of complaining less and praying more because it was through prayers that I found the strength and courage to live moment by moment, event by event, and day by day. Before I knew it, Nathan had turned eight, then twelve, sixteen, and now he's nineteen. Those words, spoken into my spirit more than a decade ago, served as a guiding light, sustaining my resolve to keep moving forward, even during times when I felt like giving up and quitting.

A second takeaway is that the symbol of the cross-shaped scar on Nathan's stomach holds a deeply personal and unique significance for him and our family. It is a source of inspiration, faith, and hope for our journey together—a symbol of God's presence and protection in Nathan's life. This scar speaks volumes about Nathan's strength and bravery in facing the challenges of his surgeries and diagnosis, a visible testament to his ability to conquer adversity.

Furthermore, the cross embodies our family's unity and unwavering support for Nathan and each other. Additionally, it serves as a profound symbol of healing and renewal, signifying our hope for a brighter and healthier future. A future where, in the presence of the Lord, all distinctions between abilities and disabilities will vanish. This emblem is a potent representation of our faith, a perpetual reminder of the remarkable journey God has guided us on and the incredible work He has accomplished in us and through us.

EPILOGUE

One of the many important lessons that life has taught me is its constant uncertainty. Life has this unique way of leading us down paths we could never have imagined. If someone had told me that I would become intimately familiar with the word "disability" and that it would shape my life's trajectory or that I would discover joy, blessings, hope, and purpose in raising a child with disabilities, I would have found it hard to believe.

At the outset, the word "disability" evoked fear and discomfort within me. It stirred unease and anxiety when I confronted it head-on, for it challenged my own beliefs and expectations. Initially, my perspective was clouded by a focus on the negatives: mourning the loss of certain expectations for a "typical" childhood and apprehension about society's perception and treatment of my son due to his disability. I also harbored concerns about potential stigmatization and his exclusion from social activities. Worries about his future, especially the limitations his disabilities may impose, weighed heavily on my mind. The financial strain required to meet his needs was a constant concern for our family. Navigating his complex requirements left me grappling with stress, exhaustion, and burnout.

I fretted about his educational prospects, future employment, and prospects for independent living. At times, I felt isolated and unsupported, exacerbated by limited access to resources, information, and a network of fellow parents grappling with similar challenges. The unpredictable (and unknown) challenges that would result because of his special needs cast a shadow of uncertainty. It left me afraid about what the future held for him and how best to plan for it.

For a while, it felt like I was walking through a thick cloud of darkness, with no idea of which way to turn or what to do. Suddenly, the clear path I once believed I was destined to follow was gone, and I was faced with something new, something different, that I didn't understand. My faith in God was what kept me going. I knew that He intimately knew the path I was meant to take because, as the scripture says, He wrote down every last one of our days, including mine, Nathan's, and each of my family members', before the first one came into being.[42] So, though I didn't know or understand where He was taking me, I trusted Him.

As I would soon come to realize, God had meticulously laid out this new path for me, complete with directional signage, well-placed rest stops, signposts, and compassionate guides. Looking back, I saw how God, the author and perfector of our faith, had been shaping and preparing me from the very beginning.

My life experiences had infused me with values and skills that would prove invaluable for advocacy. My upbringing instilled in me a strong work ethic, industriousness, responsibility, and a profound curiosity—all of which played a crucial role in establishing a movement aimed at amplifying the voices of children with disabilities and their families. My aptitude for writing and public speaking had been honed since an early age, nurtured through active participation in the debate club and involvement in local service organizations like the school-based Red Cross and my church.

Moreover, my educational background in business and my professional experiences converged seamlessly with these di-

---

42 Paraphrased from Psalm 139:16 (NIV)

verse elements, propelling me forward in my journey of raising my child and expanding my work in advocacy.

I came to truly understand the depth of the scripture: "You hem me in behind and before, and you lay your hand upon me."[43] This verse came alive for me as I realized that being "hemmed in" by God means His presence surrounds us, shielding and guiding us. It wasn't that He didn't want to support me; rather, He desired for me to cultivate the habit of turning to Him first rather than as a last resort.

As a dear friend often reminds me, as we journey through life, we are essentially "making it up as we go along." Yet, with God, who knows our end from the beginning, serving as our guiding light, who could be better to direct my steps? It was this realization that led me to delve into the Bible. And in doing so, I uncovered a wellspring of grace, strength, encouragement, hope, and guidance.

One particular verse that became foundational in my daily life and journey is Jeremiah 29:11 (NIV), which reads, "'For I know the plans I have for you,' declares the Lord, 'plans to prosper you and not to harm you, plans to give you hope and a future.'" I held onto this verse tightly during the turbulent moments of Nathan's childhood when it felt like I was sinking. Even though there were times when I couldn't personally apply this promise to myself and my son, the recurring theme in the Bible that emphasizes God's knowledge of the future and His divine plan for each individual's life served as a steady anchor.

I want to acknowledge that it's undeniable that our lives have been far from easy due to Nathan's diagnosis. Watching his battle

---

43 Psalm 139:5 (NIV)

for survival, which began even before his birth, and seeing the visible scars of his cerebral palsy has been incredibly soul-crushing. There have been numerous moments when I felt like there was no recovery from these setbacks. No matter how hard I tried, how many affirmations and declarations I made, or how fervently I bargained, I still couldn't see a way forward. Many sleepless nights were spent wondering how we could ever emerge from the abyss of debt, scarcity, and unmet needs that had engulfed us.

However, as I leaned into God, He provided me with sustenance. He unveiled doors I hadn't even known existed. He introduced me to an extraordinary global community of supporters, encouragers, mentors, teachers, and friends, some of whom you've encountered within the pages of this book. When I reflect on all of these blessings, it becomes evident that I would never have crossed paths with them or had the opportunity to know them if it weren't for Nathan and his unique gift of cerebral palsy.

People sometimes asked me what lessons I would share if I could write a letter to my younger self. I certainly wish I had some antecedent literature like this book, which would have given me an insight into the journey and what to do. I would tell my younger self that as the God-assigned parent and caretaker for this child with cerebral palsy (CP), I have been given the power to envision a bright and meaningful future for him, just like any other parent. His life would unfold differently, and his specific goals and aspirations would vary in response to his unique abilities and needs.

Today, at the age of nineteen, Nathan faces developmental delays relative to his peers in various areas, such as intellectual, academic, language, social, physical/sensory, and behavioral skills. Due to his multiple disabilities, he requires intensive support and benefits from low student-staff ratios in his programs. Nevertheless, he shines as a source of light, inspiration, and joy in our lives. Neither I nor my family members nor anyone who has met him can imagine a life without him.

Each day, as I put him on the school bus, I witness the joy in the faces of the driver and the aide as they welcome him aboard. When I attend parent conferences, I hear everyone talking about how his light shines brilliantly into their day. As I eagerly wait for his bus to arrive each afternoon, I feel light in my steps. Despite our challenges, I would willingly endure it all over again just for the immeasurable joy Nathan brings into our lives.

I wish I could reconnect with the surgeon who had performed his first surgery. I longed to show her Nathan and, in doing so, ignite the same hope in her heart that Nathan continually sparks in us and everyone he encounters. I would also tell her how damaging it is to give the parents of a three-day-old baby a fifty-fifty chance of surviving infancy or childhood. *What would have become of him had we accepted that prognosis as inevitable?*

Today, I find myself wishing for the opportunity to sit down with my younger self and reassure her that everything would ultimately be okay. If I could offer advice to the version of me just after Nathan's diagnosis, here are some of the things I would convey.

Dear Younger Self,

I know you're scared and overwhelmed right now, facing what seems like insurmountable challenges. But understand that these difficulties, though tough, will shape your life positively. Nathan's diagnosis isn't the end; it's a new beginning to a significant journey.

Keep your focus on the Lord; He'll give you big dreams for him. Pay attention to Nathan's holistic development—physical, occupational, communication, spiritual, social, and psychological. Everything you need will come, and the right people will show up.

Don't forget your family. They're crucial, and this journey will transform them as much as you and Nathan. Your voice holds significant value, so don't hesitate to express yourself. Raising Nathan will also bestow within you the ability to see and nurture each of your children's unique gifts and abilities.

You have an exceptional support network—your "village"—who will always be there when you need them. They will be the ones to lift your spirits, pray with you, offer encouragement, provide motivation, and guide you along your life's purpose. Among them, you'll find some who will become your dearest friends.

Your voice is a powerful tool for expressing your thoughts, emotions, and viewpoints. It advocates not only for Nathan but also for others. Trust in the power of your own voice, for it has the capacity to uplift and inspire.

Familiarize yourself with the concept of "collaboration" from the outset. It's required to work effectively with the diverse professionals who will provide services for Nathan. At the beginning of each collaboration, emphasize the importance of open communication, compassion, and empathy in your interactions. You'll find that many of these professionals will highly value your input and be eager to teach you what you need to know to become a more effective mother and advocate.

Set ambitious goals for Nathan's future, and never let your own (or anyone's) limitations hinder his potential. Look beyond your own limitations (and his), and instead, envision the grander plan that God has for him. Be purposeful and intentional in your actions, nurturing his growth and development to help him achieve his fullest potential.

Utilize your voice within your Christian community. It holds the power to foster understanding and compassion. Share Nathan's story and his specific needs, guiding your fellow believers toward creating more inclusive programs. Your voice is a catalyst for positive change within your community.

Ultimately, remember this: You are inherently destined for success. You possess the spirit of an overcomer, capable of enduring any challenge. Worry less, play more, laugh more, incorporate self-care, and trust in God more. Because, despite how things appear, things will get much better. There is a purposeful and remarkable future ahead of you. I give you my word on that. Your journey is replete with its own unique beauty, and the horizon promises boundless growth, enduring strength, and an abundance of empathy that will enrich your path ahead.

As I've come to realize, God sends His blessings in so many different ways. Sometimes, we might not even notice them because they don't come packaged the way we expect them to. His blessings are like hidden gems, waiting to be discovered in the most unexpected places and moments. They often arrive in the small, everyday details, the challenges that test our strength, and the people who come into our lives when we least expect it. To fully embrace these blessings, we need to keep our hearts open, ready to see the extraordinary within the ordinary.

The End

ABOUT THE AUTHOR

Christine Staple Ebanks is a distinguished author, dynamic speaker, and unwavering advocate for children with disabilities. Her remarkable journey into the world of disability advocacy began in 2005 when her son Nathan was diagnosed with cerebral palsy. The challenges she and her family encountered in accessing support and essential services for her son ignited a deep-seated passion within her to lend a voice and shine a light on the issues faced by children with disabilities and families. Her dedication extends to collaborating with families, caregivers, and communities to make the inclusion of children with disabilities in all aspects of life more meaningful.

Christine's unique perspective on raising a child with cerebral palsy spans two vastly different environments: Jamaica, where resources for children with disabilities are limited, and the United States, where parents must navigate complex systems to secure the best possible support for their children. Her dual experiences have cultivated a deep commitment to fostering inclusive environments and building robust support systems for special needs children.

At the forefront of her advocacy efforts stand two organizations she founded, the Nathan Ebanks Foundation (NEF) and Raising Special Needs Inc. (RSN). For more than a decade, her work has provided invaluable resources and support to families while advocating for policy changes that enhance the lives of special needs children. Christine's dedication extends to the professional sphere, where she actively works to build the capacity of teachers and other professionals to impact the lives of children with special needs positively.

Christine shares her insights and expertise with a wide audience through her contributions to publications like *Human Services Today*, a publication of the National Organization for Human Services Professionals, and *Accessibility Journeys* magazine, a consumer publication that showcases accessible travel possibilities and best practices. In addition to her writing, Christine actively participates in various boards and committees where her voice plays a significant role in shaping policies and practices to enhance the inclusion of children with disabilities and support their families. She is a member of the Special Education Parent Advisory Committee (SEPAC) in Somerset County, New Jersey, USA, and a former member of the National Disability Advisory Board in Jamaica.

Outside her professional commitments, Christine treasures her personal interests. She finds solace and inspiration in spending quality time with her family, nurturing her faith, reading, and taking long walks in nature. Her guiding philosophy is encapsulated in the words of Desmond Green, "while we may not be responsible for the state in which we find the world, we cannot deny our responsibility for how we leave it to those who follow in our footsteps" (Visions of Jamaica, 2010). Christine Staple Ebanks exemplifies this ethos through her unwavering dedication to improving the lives of children with disabilities and leaving a lasting legacy of inclusivity and support for future generations.